THE TRUTH ABC
A DOCUMENTED, SCIENTIFICALLY ACCURATE BOOK
BY PROFESSOR JACK A. BATEMAN

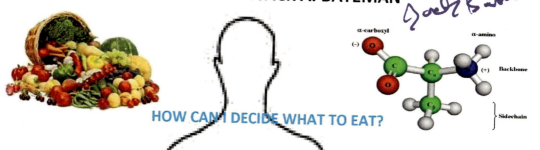

HOW CAN I DECIDE WHAT TO EAT?

HOW MUCH COENZYME Q DO I NEED?

CAN MAGNESIUM HELP MY HEART?

WHAT CAN KEEP MY LIVER HEALTHY?

HOW CAN I PREVENT COLON CANCER?

HOW CAN KEEP MY ENERGY LEVEL HIGH?

HOW CAN I BELIEVE WHAT I READ IN MAGAZINES AND NEWPAPERS?

WHY DO I NEED TO TAKE VITAMIN SUPPLEMENTS?

HOW CAN I KEEP MY IMMUNE SYSTEM OPTIMIZED?

HOW CAN I AVOID HEART DISEASE, DIABETES AND CANCER?

Table of Contents

CHAPTER 1 - HOW DID WE GET HERE? 1

CHAPTER 2 – CARBOHYDRATES 12

CHAPTER 3 - LIPIDS 23

CHAPTER 4 - PROTEIN 33

CHAPTER 5 - DIGESTION 47

CHAPTER 6 - METABOLISM 60

CHAPTER 7 - METABOLISM AT WORK: CARBOHYDRATES 70

CHAPTER 8 - METABOLISM AT WORK: LIPIDS 87

CHAPTER 9 - METABOLISM AT WORK: PROTEINS 96

CHAPTER 10 - NUTRITIONAL SUPPLEMENTS 101

CHAPTER 11 - BOGUS NUTRITION: A DISCUSSION OF CONTROVERSES 111

MENUS - EATING BY THE MEDITERRANEAN PYRAMID .... **Error! Bookmark not defined.**

INDEX 137

PREFACE - THE TRUTH ABOUT NUTRITION

The author of this book is a retired college professor of science who taught the "science of nutrition" for 30 years. He also had medical training as a licensed Medical Technologist, performing numerous laboratory tests on real people. Many of the students he taught vigorously encouraged him to write this book. He was offered to coauthor a book with his Cardiologist, Dr. Michael Ozner, later wrote his own books and become a member of the Board of Directors for the journal of Life Extension.

For six years Professor Bateman was an active member of the North American Association for Nutrition and Preventive Medicine. He was trained in molecular nutrition by Dr. Kenneth Pelletier, currently at the University of Arizona, college of medicine. Dr. Leo Galand, practicing physician in New York, City, taught him molecular metabolism of fatty acid and the necessary balance between omega 6 and omega 3 fatty acids. In 2000 he wrote a book to help his students navigate his nutrition course, Bateman, Jack, Supplement to Human Nutrition, Kendall/Hunt Publishing Company. 2000.

During his tenure at Miami-Dade College he received outstanding teaching awards five times. His diverse interests took him into the field of Biotechnology (Gene science). He was trained in Biotechnology at the Center for Biotechnology at the University of Florida. For several years, he taught Biotechnology at Miami-Dade College and the University of Miami.

After retirement in 2004, he had some health problems that side tracked his interest in science, but having regained his health after 2006, he began to focus on his love for nutrition and biotechnology. He e-published numerous articles and blogs in nutrition. He now has a modest biotechnology laboratory in his home, where he teaches young and old the magical techniques of the discipline.

He never stopped his love of nutrition. He has professed health and wellness through nutrition, exercise, and faith to most of his friends and family. His often-gentle teaching methods have changed the lives of a many.

Now, after 12 years of retirement, a passionate fire was ignited by the encouragement of friends and his endlessly loving wife, Marji to write this book. His goal is to present nutrition in a gentle, but scientifically accurate, comprehensive manner so that the reader can feel the passion for the subject.

CHAPTER 1 - HOW DID WE GET HERE?

This is not just another book about nutrition. During 30 years of teaching nutrition, a vast amount of information got stored in this author's brain. As I enter my eightieth decade of life, I am overwhelmed with the desire to share my knowledge. Since I no longer have the hundreds of students with whom I can share my knowledge, writing this book was a no brainer.

As humans evolved on this planet, they hunted for food aimlessly. When a food supply was found, they gathered all they could carry at the time. Once the food was gone, they would wander on in search of other foods. Occasionally, they were fortunate enough to happen upon an animal that was either injured or unaware of their presence, whereupon the animal would be slain for a feast. Much of the time these primitive humans were experiencing near starvation as a rule. These nomads would eat plant leaves, stems and roots along with fruits, nuts, and seeds as their primary diet.[1] Eventually, some of them got the bright idea to stay in one place and plant some of the seeds that they gathered so they could grow more food. This was the beginning of farming.

For centuries, a farm fresh food supply was available to most people. As the Industrial Revolution began, people began to cluster around a central employer; the need for foods with longer shelf lives arose. Food processing was created and the genesis of <u>factory foods</u> began. Processed foods lost nutrients, so the nutritional quality of the food supply declined. Thus, people began to show symptoms of nutrient deficiencies, which lead to degenerative diseases. As scientific medical technology, advanced, human testing for nutrients in the blood stream became available. Scientific research on animals showed clearly that certain nutrient deficiencies correlated with specific diseases.[2,3]

Why is there such deception and controversy about nutrition? Every person must eat and food choices are abundant. Most people do not know the basic principles of nutrition, or the consequences of poor food choices. These consequences are not the result of what you eat one day, but what you eat day after day over weeks and months. Eating should be a joyous event in our daily lives, complete with conversation and laughter. Many people

---

[1] Tarantino, et al. "Hype or reality: should patients with metabolic syndrome-related NAFLSD be on the Hunter-Gatherer (Paleo) diet to decrease morbidity?" Journal of Gastrointestinal and Liver Diseases, 24·35968. 2014.
[2] Williams, Roger. <u>Nutrition Against Disease.</u> Pitman. 1971
[3] Davis, Adele. <u>Let's Get Well.</u> Signet. 1965

today do not have or take the time to enjoy food. The pressures of a financially productive life have relegated food to a bothersome necessity. This hurried life-style produces stress hormones that increase metabolic chemical reactions in the body. This results in an over production of *free radicals* (molecules with unpaired electrons) that attack cell membranes, functioning proteins, mitochondria, and the genes in the nucleus. The result is that the organs in the body get constant damage that impairs their normal function.

Let's compare two lunches that a busy professional might choose. A fast food lunch of a cheeseburger, French fries, and a milk shake; verses a piece of fresh fish, broccoli, and a serving of black beans and brown rice. See the table below:

TABLE 1 - LUNCH FOOD COMPARISON

CHEESEBURGER, FRIES & MILK SHAKE		FISH, BROCCOLI, BLACK BEAN/RICE	
CALORIES	873	CALORIES	334
PROTEIN	31 g 14%	PROTEIN	25.5 g 30%
CARBOHYDRATE	124 g 57%	CARBOHYDRATE	47 g 56%
FIBER	5 g	FIBER	11 g
FAT	29 g 30%	FAT	5.4 g 14.6%
CALCIUM	515 mg	CALCIUM	98 mg
POTASSIUM	1293 mg	POTASSIUM	824 mg
SODIUM	1142 mg	SODIUM	97 mg
FOLACIN B-9	50 mg	FOLACIN B-9	181 mg
VITAMIN C	13	VITAMIN C	58 mg

today we have the luxury of scientific research around the world studying the intricate interactions between food consumption and disease. We will explore many of these scientific finding in the chapters to follow. One of the premier researchers in nutrition is Dr. Walter Willet at Harvard University.[4] His team of scientists has recently revised the *Food Pyramid* shown here.   [4] Willet, Walter. "Healthy Eating Pyramid." The Nutrition Source, Harvard T.H. Chan School of Public Health. 2016.

The Truth About Nutrition

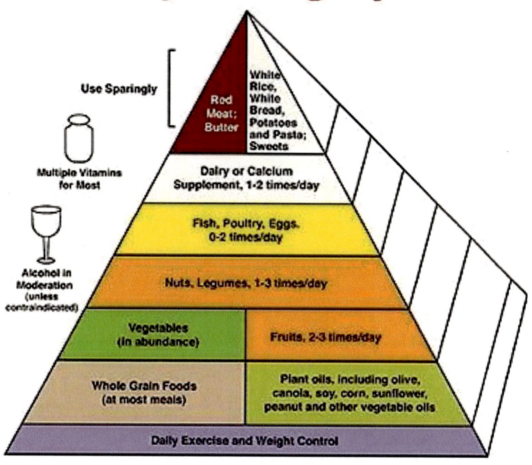

You can observe that the bottom rung of the pyramid represents EXERCISE as the most import part of anyone's daily activity. The next three rungs are all plant foods, primarily in their whole, natural state. Note that the fifth rung is the first appearance of animal protein including fish, poultry, and eggs. Where is the *beef?* It appears in the very top of the pyramid as "use sparingly". That typically means once a week. Most Americans eat beef or pork, white rice or pasta, potatoes, and desserts at most meals. These should only be eaten sparingly according to the new Willet pyramid.

Let's contrast this pyramid to the Mediterranean Pyramid. There are obvious similarities, daily exercise being the base. The whole grain foods in the second rung are much more

The Truth About Nutrition

explicit in the Mediterranean Pyramid. The daily consumption of fruits, vegetables, nuts, and legumes (beans) are similar. The addition of cheese and yogurt daily is different. The consumption of seafood, poultry and eggs are reduced to weekly along with sweets

MEDITERRANEAN PYRAMID

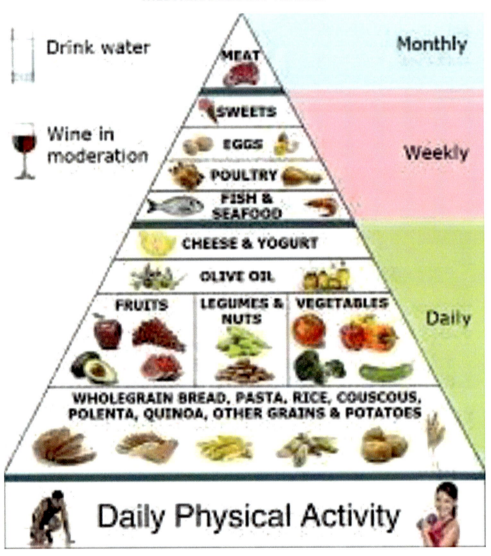

Meat is relegated to monthly. Both pyramids recommend *wine* consumption in moderation. In addition, the Willet pyramid includes a multiple vitamin; something that the American Medical Association has argued against forever. Note that only olive oil is recommended, whereas the Willet version includes several different oils. Further

The Truth About Nutrition

investigation reveals that **Extra Virgin Olive Oil** is the number one choice. But be careful, research has shown that most of the extra virgin olive oils sold in the supermarket are seriously adulterated.[5] Researchers at the University of California (Davis) found that 73% of imported and domestic brands of extra virgin olive oil were bogus.[5] Extra virgin olive oil is less refined and typically cold pressed from the olives.

Researchers have proven that the unusual benefits of consuming extra virgin olive oil are not the oil itself, but a group of compounds found in the oil called *polyphenols*. These compounds have multiple effects on cellular health including powerful antioxidant protection, antiaging, and potent gene control.[5]

[5]Downey, M. "Is Your Olive Oil Counterfeit?" Life Extension Journal. 22; 22-30. September 2016

The recommendation of wine consumption has been researched thoroughly worldwide. It was first noticed that the French consumed a higher fat diet than the typical American, yet their incidence of fatal heart attacks was much less. The difference turned out to be wine. One of the principal substances in red wine is called **Resveratrol.** There are 4079 research papers in the National Library of Medicine on Resveratrol. This author has written the article that follows:

Prevent Premature Death
The red wine and the antioxidant, resveratrol connection.
By Jack Bateman, professor of nutrition

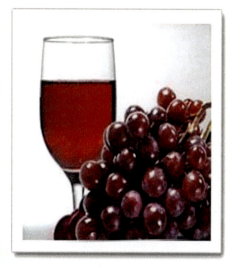

" Red, red wine you make me feel so fine" are the words of a popular song, but research is showing that the red wine may also be a life saver. It has been proven that the skin of red grapes contains chemicals called, polyphenols, that are powerful antioxidants.[1] One of those substances, resveratrol, has been isolated and purified. It is now on the market as a nutritional supplement.

The United States Department of Health and Human Services has recommended the moderate consumption of alcohol in their disease prevention Initiative publication, Healthy People 2010. There is a significant difference between consuming alcohol from beer or liquor and red wine. Research has

The Truth About Nutrition

proven that moderate alcohol consumption from any source can increase blood levels of HDL (High Density Lipoprotein). Consumption of red wine has many additional benefits. It has long been known that a high dietary fat consumption, especially saturated fat (red meat, dairy) is positively linked to CAD, coronary arterial disease, and heart attack death.[2] Paradoxically, the French diet is rich in saturated fatty foods, yet they have a low incidence of heart disease.[3] The Copenhagen Heart Study showed that wine drinkers had lower risk of CAD.[4]

The polyphenolic compounds in red wine act as antioxidants in the blood stream. Some signal the relaxation of arterial muscles, which lowers blood pressure, a causative factor in heart disease. Others neutralize free radicals, thus preventing the oxidation of Low Density Lipoproteins (LDL's), a key player in the etiology (medical cause) of atherosclerosis (the cause of CAD).[5] When oxidation of LDL occurs it damages the molecule making it toxic to the cell.

Cholesterol is very insoluble in water; thus, it is transported through the blood stream in two complex forms, LDL and HDL. LDL is commonly known as the "Bad Guy Cholesterol" and HDL is known as the "Good Guy Cholesterol". The moderate consumption of red wine has been shown to decrease the LDL and increase HDL. Furthermore, it has also been shown to decrease the oxidation of LDL.

Platelets are small cells in the blood that are essential in the regulation of blood clotting. When the platelets experience oxidative damage, they stick together, which causes a <u>blood</u> clot. Blood clots can cause a heart attack and stroke. Resveratrol, one of the polyphenols in red wine (cartoon to the left) works with vitamin E to help prevent this platelet oxidation, even in an elevated oxidative stress environment.[1] An elevated oxidative environment is one in which there is an abundance of active oxygen species, some being free radicals that can attack and damage anything. The molecule to the left is the active "trans" form of the molecule. It is found in the skin of red grapes.

Nitric oxide, NO, is a signaling molecule that is essential to healthy cardiovascular functioning, as well as several other normal physiologies. The polyphenols in red wine increase the production of NO, thus facilitating the maintenance of homeostasis (a stable balance) in the cardiovascular system.[1]

Although resveratrol has been studied extensively in cardiovascular disease (472 research studies to date), other studies have shown that it can reduce inflammation, protect against cancer, and decrease aging. Those topics will be discussed in a future chapter.

So, how much red wine should a person consume to obtain the protective effects? One study has shown efficacy with a consumption of about 1.5 cups or 12 ounces of wine per day. This amount would contain approximately 2 ounces of alcohol. Increases in HDL have been observed with as little as one half an ounce of alcohol from other sources. A double blind, randomized, placebo controlled study has shown that 100 – 150 mg of resveratrol supplement in the morning produced that highest blood levels. It also showed that the half-life, with repeated doses, was 2 – 5 hours, indicating that dosing should occur at least 3 times per day to optimize efficacy.[6]

AN ANONYMOUS QUOTE: **"God in his goodness sent the grapes, to cheer both great and small; little fools drink too much, and great fools not at all."**

REFERENCES:

1. Vadavalur, Ramesh, MD, et.al. "Significance of wine and resveratrol in cardiovascular disease: French paradox revisited." <u>Experimental Clinical Cardiology</u>. 2006; 11: 217-225.

2. Artaud-Wild, SM, et.al. "Differences in coronary mortality can be explained by differences in cholesterol and saturated fat intakes in 40 countries, but not in France and Finland: a paradox." <u>Circulation</u>. 1993; 88: 2771-9.

3. Renaud, S, et.al. "Wine, alcohol, platelets, and French paradox for coronary heart disease." <u>Lancet</u>. 1992; 339: 1523-6.

4. Gronback, M, et.al. "Type of alcohol and drinking pattern in 56,970 Danish men and women." <u>European Journal of Clinical Nutrition</u>. 2000; 54: 174-6.

5. Chakravarti, RN, et.al. "Atherosclerosis: its pathophysiology with special references to lipid peroxidation." <u>Applied Cardiology</u>. 1991; 6: 91-112.

6. Almeida, Luis, et.al. "Pharmcokinetic and safety profile of trans-resveratrol in a rising multiple-dose study in healthy volunteers." Molecular Nutrition and Food Research. 2009; 53: 1-9. #

Let's look at a couple of Mediterranean Pyramid daily menus, one for a woman and one for a man. The woman's menu:

TABLE 1 -   SAMPLE MENU FOR A WOMAN FOLLOWING THE MEDITERRANEAN PYRAMID

FOOD CONSUMED	AMT	CALORIES	PROTEIN grams	CARBO grams	FIBER grams	FAT grams
Egg, poached	1	74	6	1	0	5
Spinach	1 cup	54	6	10	6	0
Quinoa	1 cup	222	8.1	39.4	3.6	5.2
Bean Salad	0.5 cup	70	2	6.5	1.5	4
Bread, multigrain	2 slices	180	8	34	8	2
Cantaloupe	1 cup	97	2	23	2	1
Onion, raw	1 cup	60	2	14	2	0
Peppers, green	2 each	38	2	10	2	0
Coffee	1 cup	5	0	1	0	0
Marji's veg mix	3 Tbs	49	1.9	5.2	0	3
Carrots, raw	9 oz	93	3	21	6	0.3
Tea, brewed	3 cups	6	0	3	0	0
Jell-O	0.5 cup	5	1	0.25	0	0
Chicken, roasted	5 oz	242	43	0	0	6
Mushrooms	0.5 cup	21	2	4	2	0
Blue berries	0.5 cup	40	0.5	10	2	0.5
Ice Cream	1 scoop	140	4	27	3	1.5
TOTALS		1396	91.5 26%	209.4 60%	38.1	28.5 19%

The Truth About Nutrition

The woman's menu contains 11 servings of vegetables, 4 servings of whole grains, two servings of fruit, 2 servings of poultry, and one serving of dessert and one egg. 38 g of fiber is outstanding. The Calorie distribution is 26% protein, 60% carbohydrate, and 19% fat. This menu is consistent with the guidelines of the Mediterranean Pyramid. The man's menu:

TABLE 2 - SAMPLE MENU FOR A MAN FOLLOWING THE MEDITERRANEAN PYRAMID

FOOD CONSUMED	AMOUNT	CALORIES	PROTEIN (g)	CARBO (g)	FIBER (g)	FAT (g)
Grapefruit	Half	37	1	9	2	0
Yogurt	1 cup	250	11	47	0	3
Egg, poach	2 each	148	12	2	0	10
Lobster	4 oz	114	24	1.6	0	0.8
Banana	1	109	1	28	3	1
Apples	1	81	0	21	4	0.2
Grapes	0.5 cup	35	0	9	0	0.2
Beans, black	0.5 cup	114	8	20	7	0.3
Quinoa	1 cup	222	8	39.4	3.6	5.2
Salad, mixed	4 oz	90	2.8	17.6	2.3	2
Brussels, sp	3 oz	35	3	5	3	0
Onion, raw	0.5 each	30	1	7	1	0
Parsley	1 cup	11	1	2	1	0
Corn	3 oz	66	2	16	2	0.4
Strawberries	1 cup	43	1	10	3	1
Coffee	1 cup	10	0	2	0	0
Chicken	5 oz	386	32	12	0	22

Bread, multigrain	2 slices	180	8	34	8	2
	TOTALS	1961	115.8 23.6%	282.6 57.6%	39.9	48.1 22%

The men's menu contains 7 servings of vegetables, four servings of whole grains, 5 servings of fruit, 4 servings of animal protein (seafood, poultry and two eggs) and one serving of dairy. Almost 40 g of fiber is outstanding. The Calorie distribution in both menus is nearly perfect. This menu is consistent with the guidelines of the Mediterranean Pyramid.

In both of the menus displayed here, the Calories distribution between protein, carbohydrate and fat is ideal. In the female menu, the saturated fat content is only 20% of the total fat, were as the male menu has 25% saturated fat. Only high quality foods, according to the quality criteria in the following chapters, were included. No low quality, factory foods were included. In this fast paced, high technology world that we live in today, it is all too convenient to pick up a bag of this or a box of that to eat. Fast food restaurants have dominated the streets for years and are very successful. Because of public pressure for higher quality foods, most of the fast food restaurants have all begun to offer some fresh, higher quality foods. When I see a man in his 50's with a family die of colon cancer because he did not take the time to insist on a quality diet in his life, it is such a tragedy and a waste of a good human life. That man will not be around to see his children mature and have families of their own.

Let's contrast these menus to a typical American menu for a day.

The Menu:

3 - 4 inch Pancakes, 6 tablespoons of syrup, 2 pork sausage links, 6 oz Orange juice, 1 cup coffee, Cheeseburger, French fries, chocolate milk shake, mixed salad, Italian dressing, 2 cups of spaghetti with meat sauce, 1 slice of white bread with butter, 1 cup of whole milk, 1 slice of chocolate cake.

TABLE 3 - Macronutrient Totals for the above menu

CALORIES	PROTEIN	CARBOHYDRATE	FIBER	FAT
3054	99	439	29	106

The Calorie consumption is about 1.5 times the men's healthy menu on page 7. The is protein is 13% of the Calories, the carbohydrate is 57% and the fat is 31%. 29 grams of fiber is excellent. This Calorie distribution is high in high glycemic index carbohydrates, saturated fat and minimal in protein.

TABLE 4 - Micronutrient Totals for the typical American menu compared to RDA's in the last row.

Ca	Fe	Mg	K	Na	Zn	A	B 1	E	B 2	B 3	B 6	B 9	C
1625	19	264	5047	1782	16	1817	1.8	14.3	2.4	26	2.4	586	141
1200	15	400	3500	2400	10	900	1.2	15	1.3	16	1.3	400	90

CHAPTER 2 – CARBOHYDRATES

Carbohydrates are sugars and their complexes. Simple sugars are small, water loving molecules that provide most of the energy to cells. Cellular metabolism (biochemical activity of a cell) is very efficient and proficient at burning carbohydrate for energy. The chart below depicts the various dietary carbohydrates.

TABLE 5.   CARBOHYDRATE TYPES FOUND IN FOODS.

CARBOHYDRATE	COMPOSITION
GLUCOSE	SIMPLE, BLOOD SUGAR
FRUCTOSE	SIMPLE, FRUIT SUGAR
GALACTOSE	SIMPLE, FOUND IN LACTOSE
MALTOSE	MALT SUGAR = GLUCOSE + GLUCOSE
SUCROSE	CANE OR TABLE SUGAR= GLUCOSE + FRUCTOSE
LACTOSE	MILK SUGAR= GLUCOSE + GALACTOSE
STARCH	PLANT STORAGE PRODUCT - MANY GLUCOSE MOLECULES (POLYMER)
GLYCOGEN	ANIMAL STARCH = A POLYMER OF GLUCOSE with many branches
CELLULOSE	STRUCTURAL CARBOHDRATE OF PLANT CELL WALLS, POLYMER OF beta-GLUCOSE

Glucose is the primary energy molecule for all cells in the body. It is easily converted to carbon dioxide and water in the metabolic pathways of the cell. The energy from the glucose molecules is partially captured in the high-energy bonds of Adenosine TriPhosphate, **ATP.** ATP is the energy molecule of life. Every living thing runs on ATP. Question: "is this by coincidence?"

Most of the cells of the body have an elaborate mechanism for controlling the movement and absorption of glucose. The technical aspects of this will be discussed in the second half of the book. There are three organs in the body that receive their glucose independently of this complex mechanism. They are the brain (central nervous system), liver and kidneys. These organs will literally die without sufficient glucose. The brain needs a large and constant amount of glucose bathing its cells and the kidneys need a constant flow of glucose. The liver is clever in that it has learned to store sizeable quantities of glucose in a form called **glycogen.** Hormonally the liver helps control the amount of glucose in the blood stream. Ultimately it

The Truth About Nutrition

is the hypothalamus in brain that contains a mechanism (the glucostat) for establishing a blood glucose "SET POINT". The hormone, **insulin,** produced by the beta cells of the pancreas facilitates the uptake of glucose into most cells of the body. In the liver insulin promotes the conversion of glucose to glycogen (glycogenesis). Insulin also promotes the biosynthesis of protein (proteogenesis) and fat (lipogenesis). Obviously some kind of control is needed here to avoid growing into a giant. The control mechanisms are so complex and vast that we will discuss some of this in the last half of the book. It is a life and death necessity that we maintain a constant fasting (NPO, no food orally) blood sugar between 70 and 100 mg/dl.

Simplistically, this is controlled by insulin and a hormone called **glucagon.** When glucose begins to enter the blood, the pancreas releases insulin, which in turn turns on the glucose transport system in the cells (brain, liver and kidney excluded). As the glucose enters the liver and muscles, insulin promotes the conversion of glucose to glycogen to be stored. Excess glucose entering the liver can be converted to protein and fat. The fat can be stored in the liver or transported to adipose cells for long or short term storage. If the glucose level in the blood stream drops below

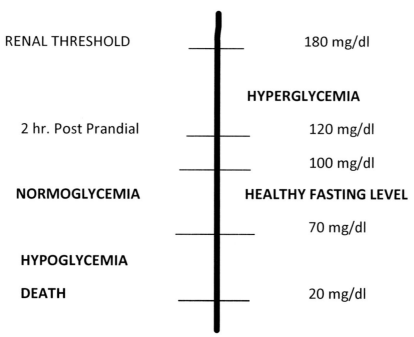

the fasting level, glucagon (think of it as "glucose is gone") is released by the alpha cells of the pancreas which tells the liver to release some of its glycogen stores.

The glucose number line represents conditions that occur at various levels of blood sugar. Normoglycemia is a blood glucose between 70 and 100 mg/dl. This is the range of normal fast blood sugar levels. After you eat a meal, your blood sugar rises, but in 2 hours after the meal (post prandial) the blood sugar level should be down to 120 mg/dl or less. In the case of Hyperglycemia (diabetes) blood sugar levels stay above 120 mg/dl. If the elevated glucose level exceeds 180 mg/dl glucose passes across the renal threshold and begins to show up in the urine. Hypoglycemia occurs when the blood sugar stays below 70 mg/dl. If it drops down to 20 mg/dl or below, DEATH can occur.

If the amounts of these hormones are controlled at normal levels **HOMEOSTASIS** occurs. Homeostasis is biological equilibrium. When homeostasis is disturbed, disease follows unless it is quickly reestablished. The muscles store glycogen, but selfishly they do not share with other cells. They can only use the glycogen for their own energy production. So, day after day, hour after hour, your blood sugar goes up and down and back up again when you eat. How does your food consumption help control this? Some carbohydrates seem to give you a rapid high, then drop you into the doldrums an hour or two later. In 1980, Professor David Jenkins at the University of Toronto created the **GLYCEMIC INDEX, GI**. This is a measure of how rapidly a measured dose of carbohydrate is absorbed into the blood stream in a given period of time. This value was determined for each food by laboratory experimentation on live humans. It has taken years and many repeat trials by many different scientists to establish the GI values in this book. It was documented that rapidly absorbed carbohydrates elicit a large insulin response into the blood stream. This results in rapid flow of glucose from the blood into the cells of the body, so much so that the blood glucose level falls below the normal fasting level. If this drop in blood sugar is more severe, it results in **HYPOGLYCEMIA** (HYPO low, GLYC glucose, EMIA in blood).

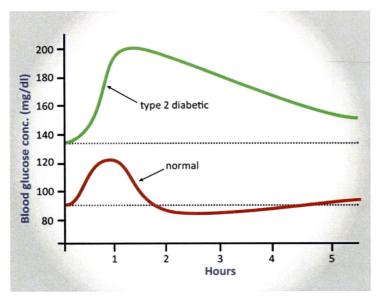

This condition comes with a well-known set of symptoms: headache, lethargy, irritability, anxiety, and/or trembling for starters. Not everyone will experience all of these symptoms at the same time and maybe never. When this happens, the symptoms can be quickly squelched by eating a carbohydrate. On the previous page is a graph of an actual glucose tolerance tests that was performed on people with varying conditions. Each curve is labeled with the person's condition. Note: in the red curve that the person started out with a fasting glucose of <100 mg/dl. Immediately there was a rapid rise in blood sugar. In one hour, their glucose peaked at about 125 mg/dl. By the end of two hours their blood glucose had dropped below their fasting level, but by the end of five hours it had slowly risen to near fasting level. This is a normal typical response to a high GI carbohydrate. Please observe that in the green curve the patient's blood sugar again rose rapidly, but did not peak until about 90 minutes into the test. At the end of five hours, their blood sugar did not drop below 155 mg/dl. This is **DIABETES.**

Below is a chart of GI values for common foods (This is not meant to be an exhaustive list.). Note that all the foods listed here contain carbohydrate.
Non-carbohydrate foods DO NOT have a GI. Low GI = 14-44. Medium GI = 45-52, High GI = 53-120 Values based on GI for Glucose = 100

TABLE 6 - GLYCEMIC INDEX

FOOD	GLYCEMIC INDEX (glucose = 100)	FOOD	GLYCEMIC INDEX (glucose = 100)
Apple, Raw	36	Mango	56
Baked Beans	40	Milk, Skim	31
Banana, Raw	48	Milk, Whole	31
Black Beans	30	Oatmeal, Old fashion	55
Blue Berries	39	Orange Juice	50
Bread, gluten free	90	Orange, Raw	45
Cake, banana	47	Peanuts	13
Cantaloupe	64	Pear, Raw	38
Carrots	39	Pineapple	66

The Truth About Nutrition

FOOD	GLYCEMIC INDEX	FOOD	GLYCEMIC INDEX
Cashews, salted	22	Pizza, cheese and tomato sauce	80
Chickpeas (garbanzos)	42	Pizza, Super Supreme	36
Chocolate, Hot	49	Pop Tarts	67
Coca cola US	63	Popcorn, microwave	55
Corn chips	42	Potato chips	56
Corn Flakes	81	Potato, Baked	111
Corn tortilla	30	Potato, mashed w butter	70
Cranberry Juice cocktail (Ocean spray)	68	Potato, sweet	70
Donut	76	Pretzels	83
Fettuccini	32	Quinoa	37
French Fries	75	Raisin Bran	61
Gatorade, orange	89	Raisins	64
Grapefruit	25	Rice Kris pies	89
Grapefruit Juice	48	Rice, Brown	68
Grapes, Black	59	Rice, White	73
Green Peas	54	Soda Crackers	74
Hamburger bun	61	Spaghetti, White	46

FOOD	GLYCEMIC INDEX	FOOD	GLYCEMIC INDEX
Honey	61	Spaghetti, Whole grain	42
Hummus	6`	Special K cereal	69
Ice Cream Regular	62	Sponge cake	46
Kidney Beans	34	Strawberries	39
Kiwifruit	52	Sucrose	64
Lentils	28	Tomato Juice	38
Lima Beans	36	Trail mix	39
Linguine	45	Vanilla wafers	77
M & M's peanut	33	Waffles, Aunt Jemima	76
Macaroni and Cheese	64	Watermelon	72
Macaroni, plain	50	White Bread	75

Since 1980, many scientists have tested food for their GI value. A comprehensive list can be found online at www.health.harvard.edu/diseases-and-conditions/the-lowdownonglycemic-index-load. A complete list of values can be found online at www.care.diabetesjournals.org/content/31/12/2281.

We can summarize the glycemic index results by performing some general observations. Observe that most fruits, legumes (beans), nuts, seeds and some whole grain products have LOW GI. These are the foods you want to concentrate on to establish a stable glucose level. When this is accomplished you will produce a stable insulin level, which is vitally important. Remember that insulin not only aids in the utilization of glucose, it also promotes the making of FAT and protein. It is the making of FAT that we want to minimize because we only make SATURATED FAT in the body. This correlates highly with the development of degenerative disease.

The Truth About Nutrition

High GI values are mostly found in foods that are highly processed, like refined grain (white flour products), factory processed foods like Pop Tarts, cakes, cookies, many cereals, white pastas, potato chips, etc.

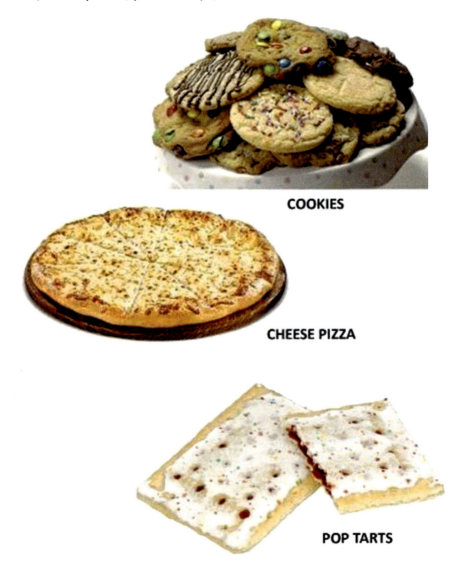

COOKIES

CHEESE PIZZA

POP TARTS

Carbohydrate foods contain complexes of sugars bonded together in different ways.

Cellulose is a type of a sugar complex composed of beta-glucose chains with many branches. We do not have digestive enzymes that allow us to utilize these fibers for energy. As they pass through the digestive tract, they scratch and tug at the internal surface of the intestines. This stimulation causes smooth muscles in the digestive tract lining to contract and relax causing the digesting food to move along down the line called peristalsis. The speed at which your swallowed food passes through the digestive tract is called **TRANSIT TIME.**

Fiber can be categorized in to *soluble and insoluble fiber.* Soluble fiber slows the transit time, but binds fats and cholesterol. Eventually these fiber bound fatty substances become feces. Soluble fiber comes from fruits called *pectin*. Plants like beans; oats and barley produce *gums, some hemicellulose and mucilage* that act as soluble fiber.

Insoluble fibers speed up the transit time by increasing the motility of the intestine. We get these from the outer coating of whole grains. Processed grains have this coating removed. Some vegetables provide insoluble fiber. This is the number one preventer of COLON CANCER! This is an insidious disease that is totally preventable.

The cartoon below graphically depicts colon cancer. Stages 1 and 2 are easily treated. Stages 3 and 4 the cancer has most likely metastasized (spread to the lymphatic system). The lights are beginning to DIM!

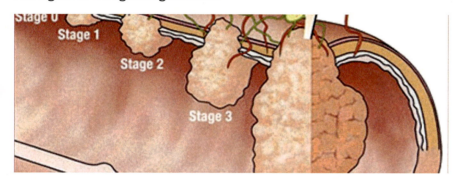

How much fiber should you have per day? The answer is 25-40 grams as a minimum. You cannot get fiber by eating meat and dairy products! You must increase your consumption of grains, fruits, and vegetables to achieve the fiber goal.

TABLE 7. FIBER CONTENT OF FOODS Adapted from: Bateman, Supplement to Human Nutrition, Kendall/Hunt Publishing. 2000.

FOOD (100g)	ENERGY (CALORIES)	CARBOHYDRATE (g)	FAT (g)	FIBER (g)	ND$_F$ x10^2
APPLES	59	15	0.5	2.8	5
AVOCADO	112	8.9	8.9	5.3	5
BLACKBERRIES	52	12.5	0.7	5.6	10
FIGS, DRIED	255	65	1	9.5	4
PRUNES, COOKED	107	28	0.4	6.5	6
RASBERRIES	49	11.4	0.8	6.5	13

The Truth About Nutrition

FOOD	CALORIES	CARBOHYDRATE	FAT	FIBER	ND
MANGO	65	17	0.5	2	3
BREAD, MULTI GRAIN	250	46	4	7.7	3
BARLEY, COOKED	123	28	0.6	3.8	3
CEREAL, ALL BRAN	258	74	3.2	32	13
GRANOLA, NATURE VALLEY	451	65	17.7	6	1
CEREAL, FRUIT'N FIBER	339	75	5.3	14	4
RICE, BROWN	111	23	1	2	2
ALMONDS	589	20	52	10.6	2
ARTICHOKE	45	9	0.6	4.8	11
BLACK BEANS	132	23	0.23	8.2	6
BROCCOLI SPEARS	28	5	0.6	2.8	10
SUNDRIED TOMATOES	257	56	3.7	13	5
SUNFLOWER SEEDS	615	14.7	58.8	5.9	0.9

Once I chaperoned a birthday party at a bowling alley. There were 20 some 5 -7year old's running around with bowling balls. Suddenly, the doors opened and this boy presents himself like he was an action hero, arms wide open and uttering some bold announcement of his arrival. He ran over to one of the bowling alleys and proceeded to charge, on foot, down the alley. He came to a sliding stop, picked himself up and ran back toward me. I gently reached out my arm and stopped him. I ask: "Excuse me, what did you have for breakfast."

He boisterously announced: "PACKMAN CEREAL" as he traveled on to join his friends. After the bowling, it was time for cake and ice cream. I glanced over at the boy's mother to discover that he was asleep on her lap. Clearly, the child was hyped up on sugar when he arrived, then after some activity he developed **hypoglycemia** and went to sleep.

Let's explore and analyze some carbohydrate meals.

DINNER MENU

Chicken breast roasted	2.5 oz	Cal= 690, Ca = 137 mg
Black Beans	0.5 cup	Prot= 48.8 g, Mg = 308 mg
Quinoa	3.5 oz	Carbs = 102 g, K = 1568 mg
Asparagus, cooked	1 cup	Fiber = 19 g, Na = 89 mg
Strawberries	1 cup	Fat= 10.3 g, B-9= 602 mg

This meal has 28% Protein, 59 % Carbohydrate, and 13 % Fat with 19 g of fiber. This is a good distribution for one meal. Recommended values are 15-20 % protein, 50 % carbohydrate, and 20-30 % fat with 25-40 g of fiber for a whole day. Average GI = 35 (low).

Let's look at a LUNCH MENU

Cantaloupe	0.5 each	Cal = 572	Ca = 161 mg
Chili w beans	1 cup	Prot = 20.8 g	Mg = 167 mg
Salad, mixed	1 cup	Carb = 67.6 g	K = 64 mg
Coffee	1 cup	Fiber = 16.3 g	Na = 1926 mg
Salad dressing	1 Tbsp	Fat = 27 g	B-9 = 87 mg
Crackers Triscuits	13 each		

This meal has 14.5 % protein, 45 % carbohydrate, and 41% fat with 16 g of fiber. Average GI = 56 (high).

A modern dietary fad is to eat a low carbohydrate diet. What happens when the body does not consume enough carbohydrate to supply the demands of the brain and kidneys? This can result in **Gluconeogenesis**. This word literally means the beginning of new glucose. Gluconeogenesis is the process of converting amino acids into glucose. In order

The Truth About Nutrition

for this to happen the nitrogen in the amino groups must be removed. The amino groups, -NH$_2$, are converted to the nitrogen waste, urea. Urea is removed from the blood stream by the kidneys. The protein breakdown to obtain the amino acid comes from muscle wasting. These are both energy demanding processes. This is not a good idea. Robbing your muscles of protein so that you can waste energy making glucose is not bright. The bottom line is that you must have a minimum amount of carbohydrate in the diet to avoid

Original Label

Nutrition Facts
Serving Size 2/3 cup (55g)
Servings Per Container About 8

Amount Per Serving
Calories 230   Calories from Fat 72

	% Daily Value*
Total Fat 8g	12%
Saturated Fat 1g	5%
Trans Fat 0g	
Cholesterol 0mg	0%
Sodium 160mg	7%
Total Carbohydrate 37g	12%
Dietary Fiber 4g	16%
Sugars 1g	
Protein 3g	
Vitamin A	10%
Vitamin C	8%
Calcium	20%
Iron	45%

* Percent Daily Values are based on a 2,000 calorie diet. Your daily value may be higher or lower depending on your calorie needs.

		Calories:	2,000	2,500
Total Fat	Less than		65g	80g
Sat Fat	Less than		20g	25g
Cholesterol	Less than		300mg	300mg
Sodium	Less than		2,400mg	2,400mg
Total Carbohydrate			300g	375g
Dietary Fiber			25g	30g

New Label

Nutrition Facts
8 servings per container
Serving size   2/3 cup (55g)

Amount per serving
Calories   **230**

	% Daily Value*
Total Fat 8g	10%
Saturated Fat 1g	5%
Trans Fat 0g	
Cholesterol 0mg	0%
Sodium 160mg	7%
Total Carbohydrate 37g	13%
Dietary Fiber 4g	14%
Total Sugars 12g	
Includes 10g Added Sugars	20%
Protein 3g	
Vitamin D 2mcg	10%
Calcium 260mg	20%
Iron 8mg	45%
Potassium 235mg	6%

* The % Daily Value (DV) tells you how much a nutrient in a serving of food contributes to a daily diet. 2,000 calories a day is used for general nutrition advice.

gluconeogenesis.

Some, so called experts, say that you need to monitor your carbohydrate intake and not the sugar intake. Carbohydrate on a food label contains the fiber, complex carbohydrate, and the sugars. The truth is that high fiber foods tend to have lower glycemic index values where as high sugar foods tend to have high GI values. Therefore, we can observe that fruits, nuts, seeds, whole grains, and legumes mostly have low GI values, even though they have high carbohydrate values. You need to consume carbohydrate sources that have low to moderate GI values. If you must eat a food with a high GI value, then eat a low GI value food along with it. Reading food labels is essential to good nutrition. The new labels will have the number of serving and the serving size prominently displayed at the top of the label. Total fat in this example is 8 g/serving with only 1 g of saturated fat and no trans-fat. This means that 7g of fat is monounsaturated and polyunsaturated fat. The total carbohydrate is 37g with 4g of fiber and 12g of sugar. This means that 21g are complex carbohydrates. The vitamins and minerals that are listed are compared to the RDA values in percentage. For example, the 8 mg of iron is 45% of the RDA based on a 2000 Calorie diet.

CHAPTER 3 - LIPIDS

Lipids are fats, oils, cholesterol, phospholipids, and sphingomyelins. These lipid molecules contain chains or rings of carbon atoms with hydrogens attached to the carbon atoms. This structure makes them very different from water molecules so that the two are incompatible. This is why fats or oils and water do not mix. Fats are composed of glycerol (3C) and one, two or three fatty acids, thus monoglyceride, diglyceride, or triglyceride.

TRIGLYCERIDE

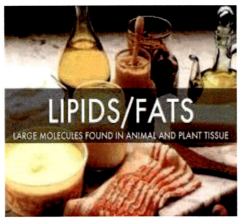

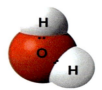

WATER

Fats are a very important source of energy for the cells, especially muscle cells. Muscle cells will preferentially burn carbohydrate because it is more efficient. Muscle cells can burn up to 60% fat with conditioning and moderate intensity exercise. Fat burning is considerably more complex than simply using carbohydrates. It is important to know that the heart burns more fat than carbohydrate because the heart never stops beating. Fat

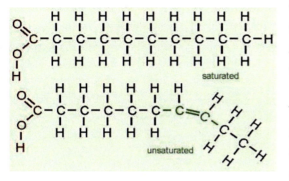

contains 2.5 times the energy content of carbohydrate. Fat contains 9 Calories per gram, whereas protein and carbohydrate contain only 4 Calories per gram.

The term *fat* is often used to describe both solid and liquid fat. Solid fat is usually what we call **saturated fat**, whereas oils are what we call **unsaturated fat.** Unfortunately, the explanation of this phenomenon is somewhat technical, so bear with me. Note in the cartoons above, the saturated fatty acid has hydrogens on every available bond whereas the unsaturated fatty acid has a double bond with two missing hydrogens and is kinked.

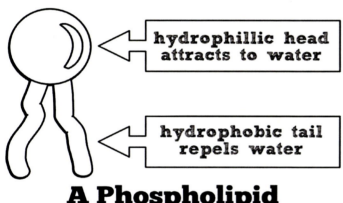

The water molecule on the last page has hydrogen atoms attached to an oxygen atom. The oxygen attracts the bonding electrons more than the hydrogen atoms, leaving the hydrogens slightly positive. Note the delta ends of the fatty acids have two oxygen atoms and a hydrogen. This end of the fatty acid is attracted to water, whereas the omega end of the hydrocarbon chain is not. Fats are mainly used in the cells to make cell membranes. The type of fat used to make cell membranes is called phospholipid. The head contains a sugar-like structure and phosphate, both of which attract water. The tails are fatty acids. They can be saturated or unsaturated. Saturated fatty acids are linear and rigid. Unsaturated fatty acids are kinked and fluid. Too much saturated fat in the cell membrane make it too rigid to be flexible, thus inhibits the proper functioning of the membrane. In the cartoon on the next page, you can observe that there are two layers of phospholipids arranged tail to tail. The phospholipids are neatly squeezed around a trans membranal protein. The protein in the membrane must move to function. In order for that to happen, the membrane must be flexible around the protein. In this cartoon, no attempt was made to differentiate saturated and unsaturated fatty acids. Note the presence of cholesterol (a very rigid molecule) between fatty acids to help stabilize them. The carbohydrate chains (green) are on the outer part of the cell membrane where they act as traffic cops. They attract and direct free moving molecules to the surface of the cell so that they can be taken into the cell. Every cell in the body contains a lot of fat in cell membranes. This is also one of the principal uses of cholesterol in the body is to stabilize the cell membrane.

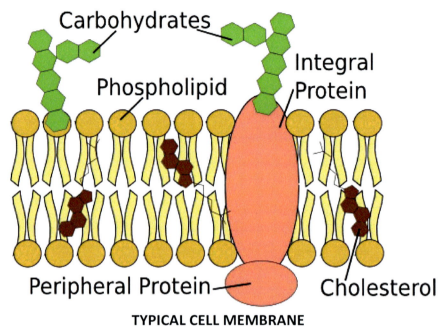

TYPICAL CELL MEMBRANE

Fat that is not being used as a functional part of the cell can be stored in adipose (fat) cells. The number of fat cells is a function of many different influences including genetics, early childhood Calorie intake, childhood obesity, adult obesity, hormone balance, etc. See the cartoon below of an adipose cell. It has a large central vesicle that can be filled up with fat.   If you consume more Calories than you use, the excess fat will be stored in adipose cells. The more you store, the more obese you become. Remember that Calories in must be equal to Calories out. Once the fat is stored it is difficult to remove.

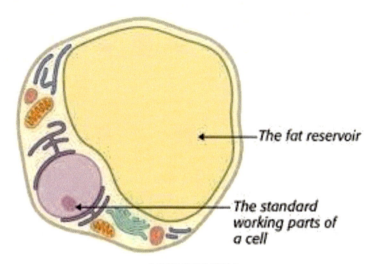

ADIPOSE CELL

Dietary consumption of fat can come from animal fat and plant fat. Red meats, duck, dairy products, palm oil and coconut oil have a high saturated fat content. For example, prime rib of beef contains 34% of its calories as saturated fat and 53%

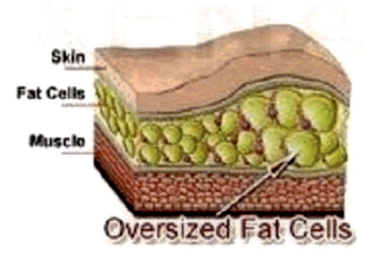

of its total Calories as fat. Coconut oil is about 90% saturated fat. Consumption of a high saturated fat diet is highly correlated with the development of degenerative diseases, heart disease and cancer. Unsaturated fatty acids include omega 9, omega 6 and omega 3 fatty acids. The sources of omega 3 fats are few and far between. Flaxseed, walnuts, and canola oil are a few sources. Some seafood sources and wild game (venison) have appreciable amounts of omega 3 fats.

Dietary sources of omega 6 polyunsaturated fats are abundant. Nuts, seed, grains, legumes (beans) and most meats are plentiful sources. The American diet is heavily skewed toward omega 6 consumption.

Omega 3 polyunsaturated fatty acids ('Ω-3PUFA'a) and omega 6 polyunsaturated fatty acids ('Ω-6PUFA) are used to make cell membranes phospholipids flexible. They are also used to make hormone-like molecules called **prostaglandins** that regulate cell processes. One of the effects of omega 6 prostaglandins is to promote inflammation. Omega 3 prostaglandins can counter this effect.

Dietary sources of omega 9 monounsaturated fats ('Ω-9MUFA) are olive oil and canola oil. Although most fats contain some omega 9 fatty acid, none match the concentration in these two sources. The cartoons below display the two fatty acids that our bodies *cannot* make and are therefore **ESSENTIAL FATTY ACIDS (EFA).** This means that the only place you can obtain them is the diet. In the first two fatty acid molecules, no attempt was made to show the altered linearity at each double C = C bond, whereas the last one, OA, displays the 45°change in linearity. The first EFA is ALA or Alpha Linolenic acid. This is an omega (Ω) 3 fatty acid since the first double bond is on the third carbon atom from the end of the molecule. The best source of this EFA is *flaxseed,* which are about 20% ALA by weight. Other sources of ALA include Canola oil (~10% by weight), Walnuts (~10% by weight), and Soybeans (~1.6% by weight). Both molecules below are bent at the double bonds making them non-linear. The second Fatty acid structure is that of Linoleic acid, the omega 6 EFA. We have a much greater risk of getting too much of this in our diets.

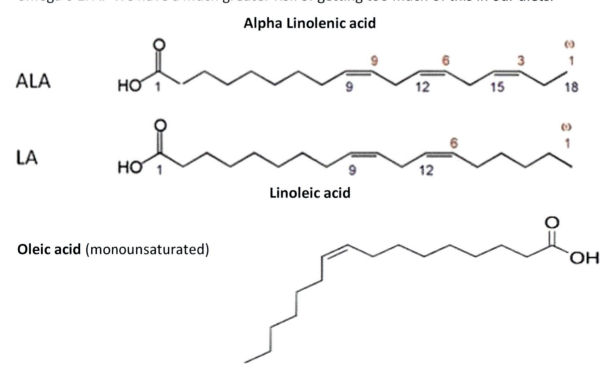

Why? The answer is because they are abundant in most of the plant fats that we eat. See the following table of oils below:

TABLE 8 - COMMON OILS USED IN THE DIET – THEIR COMPOSITION IN PERCENTS

SOURCE	TOTAL FAT (grams)	SAT. FAT %	OA % Ω-9	LA % Ω-6	ALA% Ω-3
FLAXSEED	100	11	18.5	17.3	53.2
WALNUT	100	15	13	58	14
CANOLA	100	6	58	26	10
OLIVE	100	24	78	8	0.01
CORN	100	24	25	60	0.01

Extra virgin olive oil consumption is heavily documented in medical research to promote a

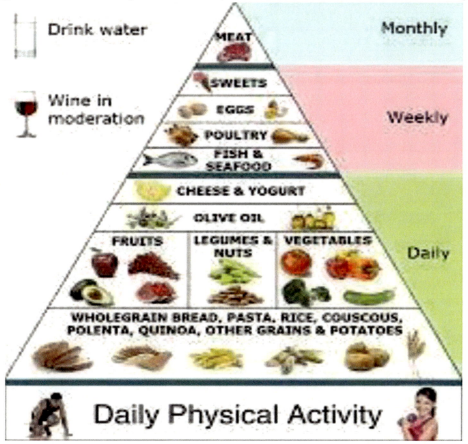

The Truth About Nutrition

healthy life in many ways. It is a mainstay in the MEDITERRANIAN DIET (see pyramid on the last page). Remember that in order to build healthy cell membranes, you need enough unsaturated fat in the diet, because cell membranes must be flexible to allow proteins to move within the membrane. Cell membranes are about 50% phospholipid and 50% protein. Your body contains over 37 Trillion cells. That takes a lot of cell membrane material. It is recommended by that American Heart Association (AHA) and the National Institute of Health (NIH) that we limit our fat consumption to between 25 – 35 % of our Calorie consumption. We should limit our consumption of *saturated fat* to 5-6 % of our fat total. Our consumption of monounsaturated fat should be around 70 %, whereas our polyunsaturated consumption should be about 24 %. That 24 % should be distributed between LA and ALA in a ratio of 6:1, minimally. (NIH)

The following table contains the fat distribution in various commonly eaten foods.

TABLE 9 - LIPID COMPARISON CHART OF A VARIETY OF FOODS (100g each). Adapted from: Bateman, **SUPPLEMENT TO HUMAN NUTRITION.** Kendall/Hunt Publishing Co. 2000

FOOD	CALORIES	T FAT g	SAT FAT g	MONO UNSAT g	POLY UNSAT g	CHOLES-TEROL mg
EGG, WHOLE	148	10	3	3.8	1.4	**426**
BUTTER	716	81	**51**	24	3	**219**
CANOLA OIL	884	100	7	59	30	0
AVOCADO FLORIDA	112	9	1.7	4.9	1.5	0
HAMBURGER MEAT ONLY 20% FAT	280	17.7	7.9	8.9	0.7	101
SALMON BROILED	216	11	1.9	5.3	2.4	87
TUNA BLUEFIN	188	5.3	1.2	1.6	1.4	38
PORK CHOP	239	13.5	5	6	1.1	80
CHICKEN BREAST	187	4.6	1.3	1.7	1.0	**202**
CHICKEN DRUM	245	14	3.7	5.5	3.7	**159**
PRIME RIB OF BEEF (LEAN)	240	14	6.2	7	0.6	81
PEANUTS	581	46	6.8	24.5	19	0

The Truth About Nutrition

FOOD	CALORIES	T FAT	SAT FAT	MONO USF	PUFA	CHOLESTEROL
ALMONDS	589	52	4.9	34	11	0.
CASHEWS	574	47	9.3	27	7.8	0
WALNUTS	607	57	3.8	12.7	37.5	0

Tuna and Salmon contain appreciable amounts of omega 3 fatty acids that are biologically active. They are the immediate precursors of omega 3 *prostaglandins* which are hormone-like molecules that help control various processes in the body, like inflammation. Remember the ALA is the essential omega 3 fatty acid. We cannot synthesize it but we can convert it into larger fatty acids that are found in the tuna and salmon. The two omega 3 fatty acids in these fish are EicosaPentenoic Acid (EPA) and DocosaHexenoic Acid (DHA). Sorry about the big scary names. It is what it is! What happens when we do not get enough of these two fatty acids? We get plenty omega 6 fatty acids. They also are used to make omega 6 prostaglandins, some of which produce inflammation. The omega 3 prostaglandins counteract this.

Please note that plant foods have no cholesterol, because only animals make cholesterol. From the table on the previous page, it is clear that butter is one of the worst culprits providing saturated fat. Remember that saturated fat is rigid. Saturated fat also has a high correlation with heart disease and cancer. Butter also has a high cholesterol. Cholesterol is not all bad. Remember that we need some to make cell membranes in our 37 Trillion cells. Cholesterol becomes a problem when we have excessive amounts of it in the blood stream. It can be exposed to oxygen and other free radicals which oxidize the cholesterol. Oxidized cholesterol is cytotoxic (toxic to cells) and sets off immune responses in the cells. White blood cells move in to feast on the toxic cells. This all leads to the disease known as **ATHEROSCLEROSIS,** the process of arterial wall damage and the accumulation of fatty plaques on the arteries. This is the beginning of CAD, coronary arterial disease. We will present technical information about atherosclerosis, heart disease, cancer, diabetes, and other degenerative diseases in the technical part of the book, if you are brave enough to venture there.

We can see from the table that egg has the highest cholesterol count of any food in the chart. On the surface this looks alarming, but research has proven over and over that the cholesterol in egg that is not fried in an iron skillet is not harmful. So, eat your eggs with confidence that they will provide you with healthy, nutritious nutrients. We will discuss this more in the PROTEIN chapter.

The Truth About Nutrition

Let's talk about **TRANS FATTY ACIDS.** This is another technical topic that is not easily explained, so bear with me. Carbon = Carbon double bonds have two hydrogen atoms, one on each carbon atom. Since the double bond restricts free rotation of the carbon atoms, the hydrogen atoms can either be on the same side or on opposite sides. In organic chemistry, the hydrogens on the same side is called *cis*. When the hydrogens are on the opposite sides, they are called *trans* (across). In nature, the normal arrangement is *cis*. This means that the fatty acid molecules will be bent at each of these C=C double bonds. Remember that this allows the cell membranes to be flexible. When unsaturated fatty acids are heated to high temperatures the molecules rearrange at these double bonds to become *trans.* This rearrangement causes the molecule to become straight like saturated fat, causing cell membranes to become rigid. This leads to premature aging and degenerative disease. The cartoon below show the comparison between *cis* and *trans* fatty acids.

CHAPTER 4 - PROTEIN

Proteins are polymers (composed of many parts) of amino acids. Human proteins are composed of 20 different amino acids, nine of which are **essential** (cannot synthesize, must be obtained in the diet). The liver can synthesize 11 of the required amino acids for the biosynthesis of protein.

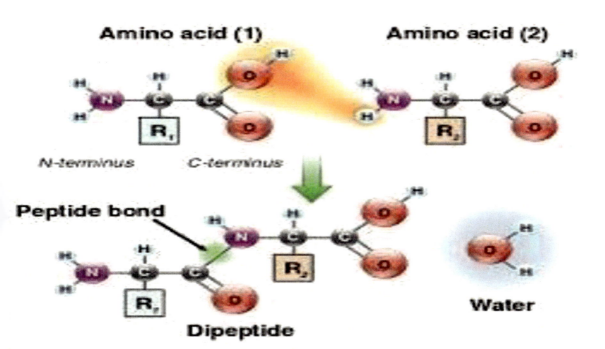

The two amino acids pictured above are combined by removing water to form a dipeptide. When this synthesis occurs over and over a polypeptide or protein is formed.
Unlike carbohydrates and fats the synthesis of protein is genetically driven via the *central dogma of DNA →mRNA →protein*. DNA = **D**eoxyribo**N**ucleic **A**cid, mRNA = messenger

RiboNucleic Acid. Every protein in your body is choreographed to perform a specific function.

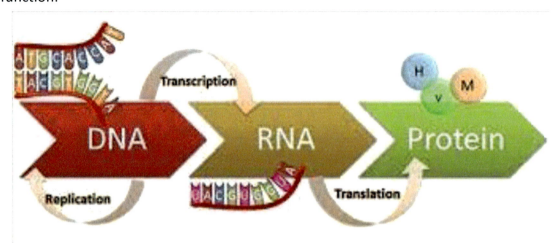

The essential amino acids include Histidine, Isoleucine, Leucine, Lysine, Methionine, Phenylalanine, Threonine, Tryptophan, and Valine.

The primary structure of proteins is a twisted linear polymer of amino acids. The secondary structure is created by the formation of bonds between amino acids stabilizing the polymer into an alpha helix. Protein polymers are then folded into a tertiary structured globular mass.   It is this final step in the activation of a protein.
Any alteration of this structure negates the function of the protein (**denaturation**). Proteins can be denatured by heat, change in pH (acidity), and reactions with free radicals or reactive chemicals.

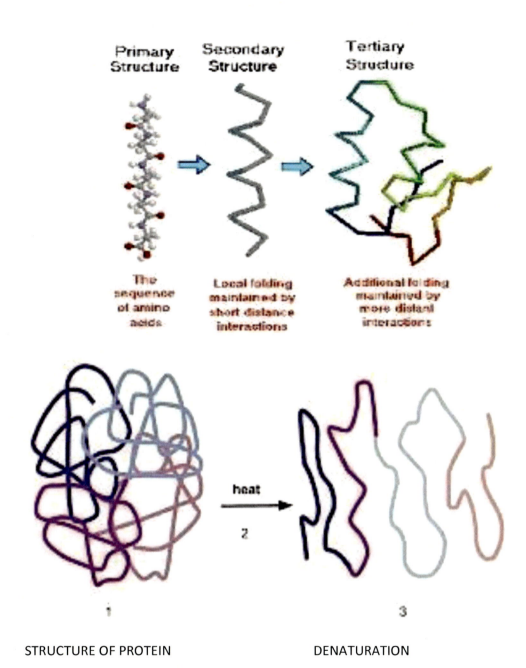

STRUCTURE OF PROTEIN

DENATURATION

Various functions of proteins are depicted in the following table.

TABLE 10 - FUNCTIONS OF PROTEIN

FUNCTIONAL PROTEINS	EXAMPLES
ENZYMES	Amylase, Sucrase, Catalase, DNA polymerase, Transferase, oxidase
HORMONES, NEUROPEPTIDES	Insulin, Glucagon, Oxytocin
CELL STRUCTURE	Keratin, Collagen
STORAGE PROTEINS	Casein, Ferritin
TRANSPORT PROTEINS	Hemoglobin, Myoglobin, Lipoproteins (HDL, LDL, VLDL)
CONTRACTILE PROTEINS	Actin, Myosin
RECEPTOR PROTEINS	Insulin receptors, LDL receptor
IMMUNOLOGICAL PROTEINS	Gamma Globulins, Interferon

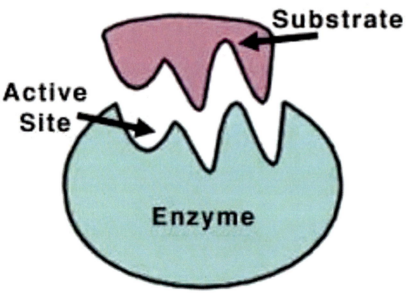

In the cartoon on the left, observe that the **Active Site** of the enzyme has a specific shape so that the **Substrate** (the molecule to be altered) can fit exactly into it.

In the **Carrier Protein** cartoon, observe that protein movement is implied in the cell membrane. The cell membrane must be flexible to allow the protein to move. The yellow spheres represent molecules to be carried across the cell membrane. The membrane must be flexible enough to allow the proteins to move.

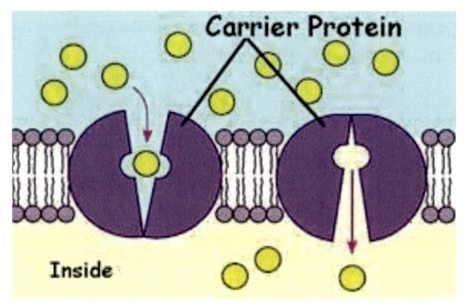

The cartoon on the next page depicts a **Receptor Site** protein that accepts a **Ligand** (a signaling molecule). Once the ligand is received, the protein moves activating a sequence of chemical events inside the cell. Remember that saturated fats, which come mostly from beef and dairy products make rigid cell membranes. This interferes with the proper movement of the membrane proteins resulting in a loss of function. This leads to degenerative disease.

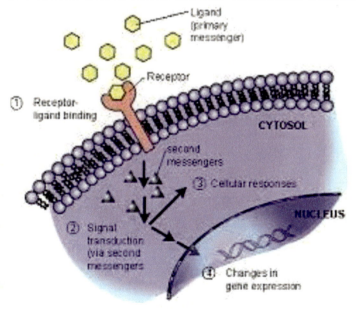

Dietary proteins come from plants and animal foods. Only animal proteins contain all 9 essential amino acids. Educated selection of plant proteins can provide all of the essential amino acids. Typically, by consuming whole grains and

The Truth About Nutrition

legumes in reasonable time proximity will accomplish this goal.

See the Table below.

TABLE 11 - PLANT PROTEIN FOOD SOURCES WITH AMINO ACID DEFICIENCIES

PLANT PROTEIN SOURCE	AMINO ACID EAA DEFICIENCY
CORN (MAIZE)	Tryptophan, Threonine
CEREAL GRAINS	Lysine
LEGUMES	Methionine, Tryptophan
PEANUTS	Methionine, Lysine
RICE	Tryptophan, Threonine
SOYBEANS, BLACK BEANS	Methionine

You can see from the table above combining plant sources of protein serves to eliminate the deficiency of an amino acid. Examples: Corn + Wheat, Corn + Black Beans, Cereal Grains + Legumes.

A vital consideration when selecting protein sources is the **protein efficiency**. This is a measure of the percentage of the consumed protein source that actually becomes human protein in your body. Of course, the most efficient sources would be eating other human beings, but this is highly illegal. Excess protein consumption means that you will have excess amino acids in the blood stream. When they are broken down in metabolism you must get rid of the nitrogen from the amino groups. Nitrogen waste compounds are all toxic. Human metabolism converts amino groups into a waste called **urea** in the urea cycle. This process requires energy and the resulting urea is toxic. The kidneys remove it from the blood and it passes out of the body as urine. The higher the percent waste, the greater the load on your kidneys and the more toxic nitrogen waste in the blood.

Consider the following protein efficiency chart:

TABLE 12 - PROTEIN EFFICIENCY

PROTEIN SOURCE	PERCENT INCORPORATION	PERCENT WASTE
EGG	94	6
MILK, COWS	82	18

The Truth About Nutrition

PROTEIN SOURCE	PERCENT INCORPORATION	PERCENT WASTE
FISH (average of seafood)	80	20
Cottage Cheese	70	30
RICE, WHOLE GRAIN	70	30
RED MEAT AND POULTRY	67	33
SOYBEANS, BLACK BEANS	61	39
WHEAT, WHOLE	60	40
CASHEWS	58	42
LIMA BEANS	52	48
CORN	51	49
WALNUTS	50	50
PEAS	47	53
KIDNEY BEANS	38	62
LENTILS	30	70
QUINOA	29	71

Suppose that your primary food source consisted of kidney beans, lentils, and quinoa. The percent of protein waste would be between 62 and 71%. Your kidneys would have to work overtime to rid your body of the urea load being produced. You only have two kidneys and you cannot live without them. Most people never think about the nutritional abuse that we unknowingly do to our bodies. So, what food choices for protein should you make?

Strangely enough the chicken egg turns out to be the most efficient protein we can eat. Unfortunately, there are few plant sources of protein that are very efficient. Our best choices for protein include EGG, DAIRY PRODUCTS, and SEAFOOD. It is wise to eat a variety of foods because each food brings a set of micronutrients (vitamins and minerals) to the party. Even though plant sources have notoriously inefficient protein, the compromise pays dividends in fiber, vitamins, minerals, and a plethora of chemical antioxidants.

The Truth About Nutrition

Next let's consider the amount of protein in a food and how many Calories it is going to cost us. Observe the Table below that concentrates on higher efficiency sources:

TABLE 13. PROTEIN IN FOOD with Nutrient Density with respect to protein times 100. (adapted from Bateman, Supplement to Human Nutrition, Kendall/Hunt Publishing. 2000.)

FOOD	AMOUNT	ENERGY CALORIES	PROTEIN grams	CARBO grams	FAT grams	CHOL mg	ND p2 X 10
Brown Rice	0.5 cup	108	2.4 9%	22.4 83%	0.8 7%	0	2.2
FOOD	AMOUNT	ENERGY CALORIES	PROTEIN grams	CARBO grams	FAT grams	CHOL mg	ND p2 X 10
Black Beans	0.5 cup	113.5	7.4 26%	20 70%	0.5 4%	0	6.5
Combined	1 cup	221.5	9.8 17%	42.4 77%	1.3 5%	0	4.4
Hamburger	3 oz	231	21.4 37%	0	16 63%	86	9.3
Beef p. rib	3 oz	319	19 24%	0	26 73%	72	6.0
Cottage cheese	3 oz	62	10.5 68%	2.3 15%	0.75 11%	3.8	17.1
Egg poached	3 oz	126	6.2 34%	1 3%	8.5 62%	212	5.0
Ham lean	3 oz	123	18 58.5	1.5 4%	4.5 33%	45	14.6
Chicken w	3 oz	145	26 71.7%	0	1.2 7%	75	17.9
FOOD	AMOUNT	ENERGY	PROTEIN	CARBO	FAT	CHOL	ND

The Truth About Nutrition

Chicken d	3 oz	173	23 53%	0	8 42%	78	13.3
Turkey w	3 oz	133	26 78%	0	1 7%	59	19.5
Milk whole	3 oz	51	2.5 19.6%	3.7 29%	2.5 44%	11	7.3
Milk skim	3 oz	29	2.5 34.5%	3.8 52%	0	1.3	13.1
Grouper	3 oz	100	22 89%	0	1.2 11%	40	22.0
Lobster	3 oz	100	22 89%	0	0.2 6%	60	22.0
Salmon	3 oz	157	24 62%	0	6.6 38%	69	15.3
Shrimp	3 oz	84	19 90%	0	0.9 10%	168	22.6

What is **NUTRIENT DENSITY (ND)?** It is a ratio of protein to Calories. Any nutrient can be substituted for protein. It is displayed symbolically as **ND$_X$** (nutrient density with respect to X) Ideally you want the most "bang for your buck", meaning that you want to get the most protein for the expenditure of the least number of Calories. Nutrient Density is a quick and easy way to make that decision. Let's observe on page 41 that there are three sources with ND of 22 or more. They are Grouper, Lobster, and Shrimp. The uninformed would quickly counter with "ah ha", there is a price to pay for eating shrimp; look at the high cholesterol. Research shows that shrimp consume a large amount of algal fiber, which is a complex carbohydrate. This fiber bonds to cholesterol, keeping you from absorbing it. (Childs) Observe that the Nutrient Density of egg is only 5 even though it is the most efficient source of protein. This is because there is not a lot of protein in egg relative to its Calorie count. Plant protein sources typically have low Nutrient Density values; however Black Beans have a higher Nutrient Density than Prime Rib. This is because Prime Rib contains a large amount of FAT.

SHRIMP

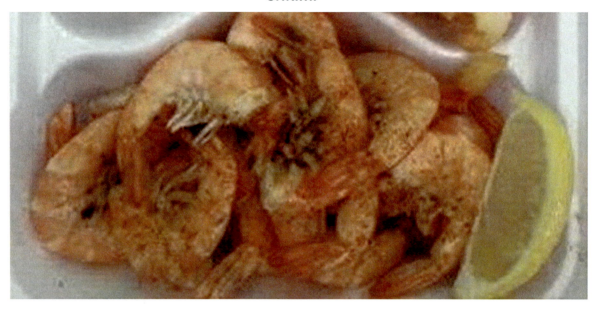

GROUPER

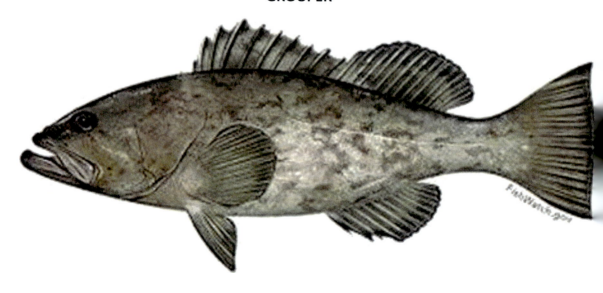

SALMON

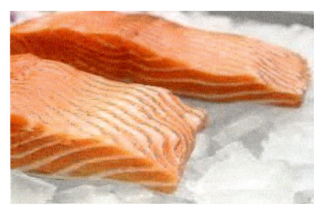

Here is some wisdom about purchasing seafood. All commercial shrimp are frozen on the ships to keep them fresh. The only time you can buy "fresh shrimp" is from a private fisherman, selling on the road-side. In the grocery, you can buy the thawed shrimp in the ice counter or you can buy them still frozen. Which one is going to be fresher? The still frozen one will be fresher. After you purchase thawed shrimp, they follow you home in a sealed package and you refrigerate them. In this thawed state, they begin to experience bacterial decomposition. The protein in seafood is very delicate in that it readily decomposes, so the longer you wait to eat them, the more decomposed they become. During the decomposition, toxic amines are formed. This is the *fishy smell* that occurs. Bad things can happen!

One of the biggest scams in seafood is the alleged serving of GROUPER in restaurants. The restaurants know that the public is will to pay extra for this delicacy, so they substitute a cheap fish for grouper and serve it to you cooked, thinking that you are too naive to know the difference. Let me educate you. Grouper is a very powerful fish. Their muscles are big and strong, which gives them a texture of a tender beef steak. Grouper substitutes are almost always a soft, mushy fish with no muscular definition or hardy texture. Coincidentally, it is against the law for restaurants to do this. As a biotechnologist, I have always wanted to develop a quick and easy test for real grouper protein, and then go around exposing these rip-off artists. Caveat emptor means, "let the buyer beware". In the grocery, you can see the muscle curves in the real grouper. They are ripped or cut up as they say in the exercise gym. I have caught and speared these fish, so let me tell you that they are strong fighters.

When you purchase fish that is thawed, you should always smell it. If there is any hint of fishiness, DO NOT BUY IT! Fish do not stink when they are fresh; they have no odor. Thawed shrimp will have a fishy odor, because they are decomposing. When any seafood decomposes, the protein begins the process of being digested by bacteria, releasing protein digestive products called amines. They all stink.

Salmon is one of the best fish you can eat. Salmon has a decent amount of omega 3 fatty acids (EPA and DHA). Wild caught salmon are ideal, but our fisheries are being depleted rapidly. Farming is the only way to go. Unfortunately, some countries do not scrutinize fish farming allowing the farmers to grow fish in unsanitary conditions. In most countries, fish are farmed near shore. These areas are exposed to street and industrial run-off water that is polluted with toxic chemical from pesticides to heavy metals. These toxins wind up in the tissues of the fish. Some areas of South America still have safe fish farming practices. I am not so sure about the Far East. A technical article will appear in a later publication.

There are many spurious claims in the popular nutrition literature. If you want to know the truth, you must go the peer reviewed scientific literature. Where do you find this? There are two sources that this author relies on: 1. PubMed.com and 2. Google Scholar.com. Often these sites only have abstracts, which are brief, introductory paragraphs that tell the reader what they did, the results, and the conclusions. In today's scientific literature you can sometimes access the entire article for free. Most of them will charge a fee of up to $40 or so.

Here are some examples of some *abstracts*:

Am J Clin Nutr. 1990 Jun;51(6):1020-7.

Effects of shellfish consumption on lipoproteins in normolipidemic men

Childs MT[1], Dorsett CS, King IB, Ostrander JG, Yamanaka WK. **Author information**

Abstract

Eighteen normolipidemic males were fed six different species of shellfish; each shellfish was fed so that protein in shellfish equaled that in animal foods in the normal diet, with less than one-half of the amount of fat in animal foods allowed for preparation of the shellfish.

Oyster, clam, crab, and mussel diets, low in cholesterol and high in n-3 fatty acids, lowered VLDL triglycerides and cholesterol and, except for the mussel diet, LDL and total cholesterol. **Squid and shrimp diets, higher in cholesterol and lower in n-3 fatty acids, did**

not change the blood lipids. The ratio of LDL to HDL cholesterol was decreased on the oyster and mussel diets. Oyster, mussel, and squid diets increased HDL2 cholesterol. Cholesterol absorption was decreased on the oyster, clam, and mussel diets. When consumed with moderate dietary fat restriction, oysters, clams, mussels, and crab appear to be useful in hypolipidemic diets for normolipidemic men. #

Biosci Biotechnol Biochem. 1998 Jul;62(7):1369-75..

Effects of dietary shrimp, squid and octopus on serum and liver lipid levels in mice.

Tanaka K[1], Sakai T, Ikeda I, Imaizumi K, Sugano M.
Author information
Abstract
The effects of three seafoods, shrimp, squid and octopus, on lipid metabolism were investigated in mice fed on 0.1% and 1.0% cholesterol-supplemented diets in the first experiment. One of each of these seafoods and casein were added to the basal diet at levels of 15% and 5%, respectively, as proteins. Casein served as the sole protein source of the control diet. **The serum cholesterol concentration was significantly lower in the mice fed on shrimp and squid in the 0.1% cholesterol diet and on any seafood in the 1.0% cholesterol diet when compared with that in the mice fed on the control diet. The liver cholesterol concentration was significantly lower in all seafood groups given the 0.1% cholesterol diet, and in the squid and octopus groups given the 1.0% cholesterol diet.** In the second experiment, the effect of these seafoods on lipid metabolism was compared with that of their defatted products in mice fed on a 0.2% cholesterol diet. Defatting resulted in an increase in the serum cholesterol and triglyceride levels in the shrimp and squid groups. The hepatic cholesterol concentration in all the seafood groups was significantly lower than that in the control group, and defatting did not influence the liver cholesterol concentration. Fecal total steroid excretion was higher in all the seafood groups when compared with that in the control group, and was not modified by the removal of fats. Thus, shrimp, squid and octopus exerted hypolipidemic activity; the serum cholesterol-lowering activity of shrimp and squid was attributed to their lipid fraction, whereas the non-lipid fraction of shrimp, squid and octopus contributed to a reduction of hepatic cholesterol and an increase of fecal steroid excretion. #

Br J Nutr. 2016 Jan 14;115(1):55-61. doi: 10.1017/S0007114515004183. Epub 2015 Nov 2.

Effect of bread gluten content on gastrointestinal function: a crossover MRI study on healthy humans.

Coletta M[1], Gates FK[2], Marciani L[3], Shiwani H[3], Major G[3], Hoad CL[4], Chaddock G[4], Gowland PA[4], Spiller RC[3].

Author information

Abstract

Gluten is a crucial functional component of bread, but the effect of increasing gluten content on gastrointestinal (GI) function remains uncertain. Our aim was to investigate the effect of increasing gluten content on GI function and symptoms in healthy participants using the unique capabilities of MRI. A total of twelve healthy participants completed this randomized, mechanistic, open-label, three-way crossover study. On days 1 and 2 they consumed either gluten-free bread (GFB), or normal gluten content bread (NGCB) or added gluten content bread (AGCB). The same bread was consumed on day 3, and MRI scans were performed every 60 min from fasting baseline up to 360 min after eating. The appearance of the gastric chime in the images was assessed using a visual heterogeneity score. Gastric volumes, the small bowel water content (SBWC), colonic volumes and colonic gas content and GI symptoms were measured. Fasting transverse colonic volume after the 2-d preload was significantly higher after GFB compared with NGCB and AGCB with a dose-dependent response (289 (SEM 96) v. 212 (SEM 74) v. 179 (SEM 87) ml, respectively; P=0·02). The intragastric chyme heterogeneity score was higher for the bread with increased gluten (AGCB 6 (interquartile range (IQR) 0·5) compared with GFB 3 (IQR 0·5); P=0·003). However, gastric half-emptying time was not different between breads nor were study day GI symptoms, postprandial SBWC, colonic volume and gas content. This MRI study showed novel mechanistic insights in the GI responses to different breads, which are poorly understood notwithstanding the importance of this staple food.

\#

One topic that you frequently see in the popular literature is that you need to eat your food as uncooked as possible to preserve the enzymes in the food, so that they can remain active in your body. All natural foods have active enzymes. Remember these are proteins that function because of their very specific shape. Heating, treatment with acids, digestive enzymes, or reactive chemicals will **denature** these proteins, thus altering their shape and function. Let me ask you, "When you eat food where do you put it"; obviously, you put it in your mouth. Then what? You chew it and swallow it, where it passes through the long tube called the esophagus and into the stomach. What happens to the food in the stomach? It is bathed in a strong acid solution, pH of about 1, along with some powerful protein digestive enzymes (proteases). Now what do you think happens to the shape of the enzymes in the food? Anyone can see that they get denatured and rendered biologically inactive. (See the cartoon "denaturation" page 35). The enzymes in fresh food do not survive that hostile environment of the stomach except for the few that are activated in an acid environment, like the enzymes in pineapple and papaya.

CHAPTER 5 - DIGESTION

When food enters the mouth, the chewing process begins along with the mixing of the food with *saliva.* Saliva is secreted by the salivary glands that are located below the lower jaw bone. Saliva is a mixture of a stringy protein called mucus, water, electrolytes, white blood cells, epithelial cells, the enzymes *Amylase* and *lingual lipase*, and antimicrobials IgA and Lysozyme. Saliva lubricates the food as it is chewed (masticated) into a food ball. Prolonged chewing allows the oral digestive process to progress. People in today's world are in such a hurry to eat that they do not chew effectively or efficiently. Oral digestion barely has time to begin before the food is swallowed. Once the food ball is swallowed, it passes down the "food tube" called the *esophagus* and into the stomach via the cardioesophageal sphincter valve. The food ball, **chyme** is immediately flooded with a stomach secretion called **gastric juice**. This digestive juice is a water mixture of hydrochloric acid, HCl (a strong acid with a pH of between 1 and 2. This acid is commonly called *muriatic acid*, sold in hardware stores for cleaning metal and adjusting the pH in swimming pools. If you would put this acid in your mouth, it would **burn** the lining of your mouth causing open sores to occur. The lining of the stomach is coated with mucus to protect it from the acid. The acid kills most microbes present in the food. Drinking superhot liquids or straight alcoholic liquors can temporarily remove the protective coating of the stomach. This allows the acid to burn the stomach.

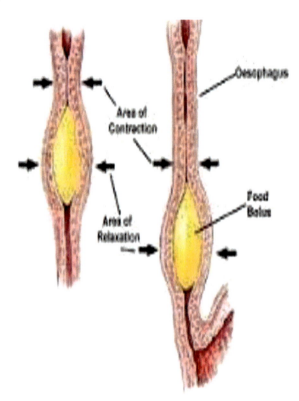

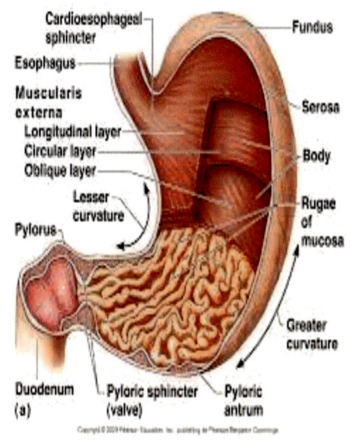

In addition to the acid, gastric juice also contains mucus, water, electrolytes (potassium and sodium chloride) and protease enzymes that digest protein. When the proteins in the chyme are bathed in acid they denature and begin to hydrolyze (break apart by adding water across the peptide bonds). The proteases (prote = protein, -ase = enzyme) continue the digestive process of breaking apart the chain of amino acids in the protein. The glands in the stomach lining secrete the HCl into the lumen of the stomach while secreting bicarbonate (a basic ion) into the blood stream. This slightly raises the pH of the blood which tends to make you sleepy. The *pyloric* value at the distil end of the stomach remains closed until the pH reaches an optimal level, then it opens while the stomach muscles contract, sending the chyme into the **duodenum.**

peptide bond is a bond between an acid group (COOH) and an amino group – NH₂). When a water molecule H-O-H is removed the peptide bond is formed. The reverse is called digestion (hydrolysis). All digestive processes are forms of hydrolysis. In the stomach, large protein chains are cleaved into smaller chains called, *peptides*. Proteins are polypeptides.

The Truth About Nutrition   49

Absorption is the process of digested nutrients passing across the membrane lining of the digestive tract. Very little absorption occurs in the stomach. Alcohol and some drugs are absorbed in the stomach.

There is a disease called **GastroEsophageal Reflux Disease or GERD (heartburn)** that over 60 million people suffer from. Once swallowed food enters the stomach, the *cardioesophageal valve* closes and is supposed to remain closed. There are several conditions that will cause it to open. One is consuming straight alcoholic beverages during a meal. Another cause is smoking during a meal. A third cause is the weakening of the valve muscle itself. A fourth cause is extreme over eating and a fifth cause is psychological stress. When the valve relaxes, the churning, acidic chyme is forced up into the esophagus. The esophagus is not equipped to support an acid attack, so the tissue begins to **burn**. Over time, day after day, week after week, the esophagus begins to wear away. The walls of the esophagus get weaker and weaker until this tissue ruptures. Now you have a *life or death* situation. Acidic food oozes out of the esophagus into the chest cavity, where a life-threatening infection begins. **NEVER LET THE BURN CONTINUE!**

There is an over **ten-billion-dollar** industry in this country that treats GERD. There are antacids that neutralize the acid. There are drugs that block the acid production in the stomach. Use the therapy that is available. Remember that all drugs have side effects. Let the buyer beware.

Another disease that is prevalent is the stomach is an infection of Helicobacter pylori. This bacteria burrow into the lining of the stomach and or the duodenum causing lesions that produce **ulcers**. This can be life threatening. Once diagnosed, it can be successfully treated with antibiotics. Untreated, this condition can lead to cancer.

Even though the gastric gland secretes an enzyme (lipase) that begins the digestion of fat the results are not very impressive. Fat is not water soluble, thus fat molecules stick together making it difficult for the lipase enzyme to access the fat molecules.   The length of time that the food remains in the stomach varies greatly with the person's genetics, the type of food consumed and the person's conditioning. Obesity tends to slow down the **transit time**, which is the time that it takes for food to pass through the digestive tract. The average time for food to stay in the stomach is between three and five hours. You can determine your personal transit time by consuming a hand full of frozen corn with a meal, after which you need to observe your stools within twelve hours until you see the corn appear. Twelve hours would be a fast transit time, longer than twentyfour hours would be an extended transit time.

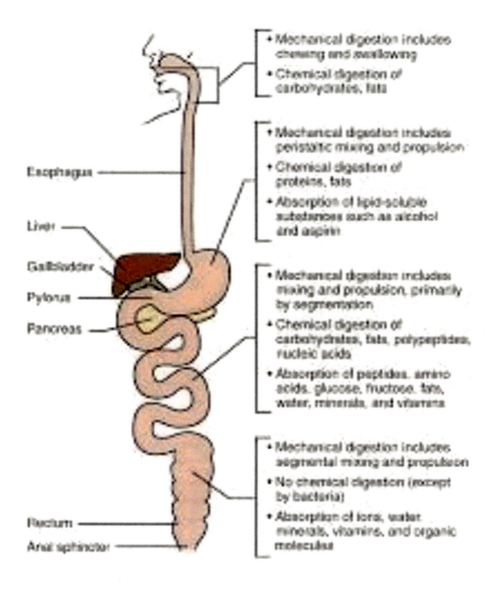

Once the chyme has had a chance to be digested and when the acidity is right, the pyloric valve opens and the food ball passes into the first segment of the small intestine called the **duodenum**. The duodenum is only about a foot long, but it is perhaps like *Grand Central Station*, in that a lot of activity occurs there in a hurry. The pancreas secretes **pancreatic juice** that contains sodium bicarbonate to neutralize the stomach acid. This often creates carbon dioxide gas that results in a belch during a meal. Pancreatic juice contains several digestive enzymes: amylase, lipase, and proteases. Amylase digests starch into maltose; a double sugar composed of two glucose molecules. Lipase digests triglycerides (fats) into monoglycerides and free fatty acids. Proteases continue the digestion of polypeptides into smaller peptides.

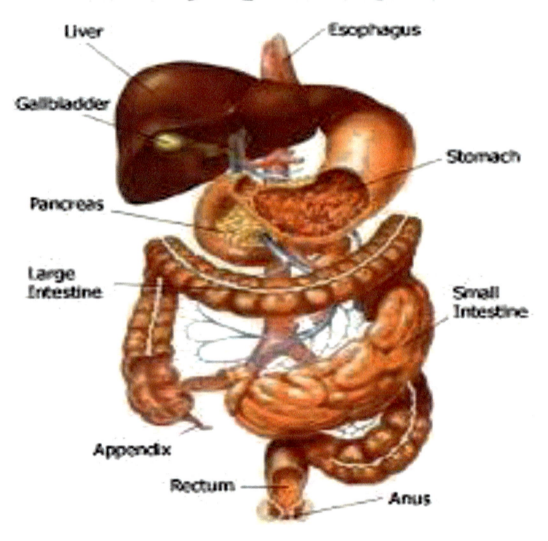

Bile is secreted from the gall bladder. The gall bladder is adherent to the underside of the liver (see cartoons below). Bile is a mixture of Cholesterol surrounded by phospholipids forming a complex called a micelle. Bile is a waste disposal system. This is the main way the body must get rid of cholesterol. The other way is exfoliation (loss of cells from the digestive tract and the respiratory tract. Bile salts are another component which are made from cholesterol acids and metal ions like calcium and sodium. Two of the wastes that provide the color of bile are the hemoglobin breakdown products, bilirubin (yellow) and biliverdin

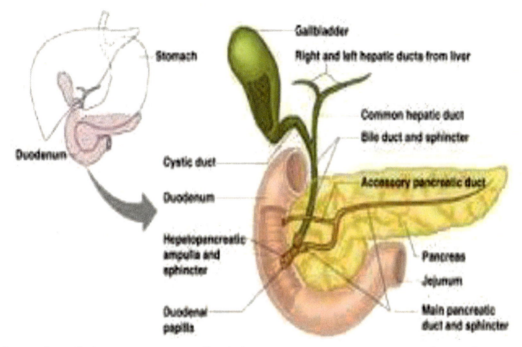

(green). Bile is a nasty tasting fluid that sometimes is regurgitated into the mouth, something that you will never forget.

Bile is the emulsifying agent for fat in the small intestine. Fats and cholesterol are problem molecules in that they are not soluble in water, so they tend to aggregate together. This is reminiscent of teenage boys at their first dance, all hovered together in one place watching the girls. Emulsification is the technical term for what a detergent does to the grease on a dirty dinner plate. In the cartoon to the below, a detergent is surrounding an oil droplet, SLS (sodium laurel sulfate). SLS is the detergent in toothpaste.

The action of the detergent allows the oil or fat to mix with water. The oil does not actually dissolve in the water. If you took a glass of water and placed a tablespoon of oil in it, there would be no mixing of the two. Now add a few drops of dish detergent and shake the glass. The oil is no longer separated. You wind up with a cloudy glass of water, because the detergent formed micelles (*my cells*) with tiny droplets of oil. This is what bile does to fats and oils in the food that we eat.

Let's explore the cholesterol dilemma.

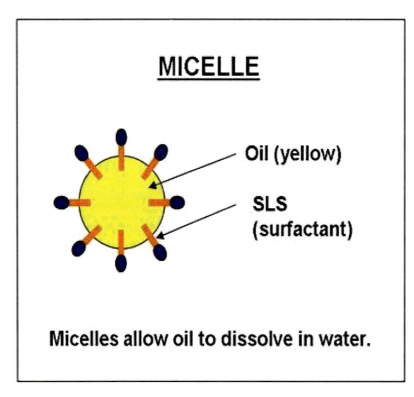

Micelles allow oil to dissolve in water.

Cholesterol is a unique molecule compared to other food molecules. We do not have the appropriate enzymes to break the ring structure shown here. We do have enzymes that can alter the carbon chain shown at the top of the molecule. This is how the liver can oxidize the end of the chain to form an acid, which in turn forms a salt. The inability to break these ring structures creates the dilemma. How do we get rid of this thing? Our amazing biochemical bodies have a rather complicated mechanism for dealing with cholesterol once it is in the blood stream. It is absorbed along with fats and oils

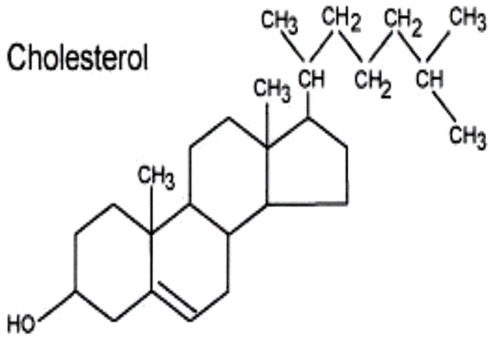

The Truth About Nutrition

(triglycerides) in the form of bile salt micelles. The bile salts are returned to the intestinal tract while the triglycerides and cholesterol are surrounded by phospholipids in the blood stream to form micelles called **chylomicrons.** The chylomicrons are transported to the liver where they are repackaged into complexes that are recognized by receptor sites on the surface of our cell membranes.   The cartoon to the left is a chylomicron We will explore this further in a later chapter.

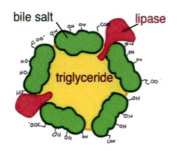

FATS & CHOLESTEROL IN FOOD → BILE MIXES WITH LIPIDS TO FORM MICELLES   LIPID MICELLES ARE ABSORBED INTO THE BLOOD → LIPIDS COMBINE WITH PHOSPHOLIPIDS TO FORM CHYLOMICRONS

What are the fates of cholesterol after it arrives in the blood stream? The liver receives most of the chylomicrons, where enzymes disassemble them. The chylomicron cartoon shows the enzyme lipase attacking the triglycerides, converting them into monoglycerides and free fatty acids. The liver repackages all the lipids into **Lipoprotein complexes,** sending them back into the blood to be transported to the cells of the body. Cells use cholesterol to make cell membranes in the cells. Some cells use cholesterol to make hormones. Excess cholesterol is transported back to the liver to be converted to bile. Bile leaves the body in the feces. A slow transit time favors the reabsorption of bile which can lead to elevated cholesterol in the blood. This reabsorbed bile is mostly oxidized which makes it extremely dangerous. Remember that "soluble" fiber from fruits and vegetables bind cholesterol. This helps send cholesterol to the toilet.

There are no valves that separate the duodenum from the next segment of the small intestine called the **jejunum**. The rhythmic contraction of the smooth muscle layers of the intestine produce a snake-like movement known as **peristalsis.** Most digestion and absorption occur in the 8-foot jejunum. The following digestive processes occur in the jejunum:

ENZYME	SUBSTRATE	ABSORPTION PRODUCT
Peptidase	Peptides →	Amino Acids
Sucrase	Sucrose →	Glucose + Fructose
Maltase	Maltose →	Glucose + Glucose
Lactase	Lactose →	Glucose + Galactose

Lecithinase Lecithin → Monoglycerides + choline + phosphate

Nucleotidase Nucleotides → Nucleoside + phosphate

The peptides are the protein digestive products of the stomach. They are digested into amino acids that are absorbed through the wall of the jejunum. Sucrose is table sugar. It is digested into glucose and fructose, two simple sugars that are absorbed in the jejunum. Maltose is malt sugar and lactose is milk sugar. They are digested into simple sugars for subsequent absorption. Lecithin is a phospholipid. Remember that phospholipids make up cell membranes, so everything that you eat that was once alive contains cell membrane material. Nucleotides make up the genetic molecules of life, so everything you eat that was once alive contain these genetic molecules. They are too large to absorb, so they must be digested into smaller components that we can use to make our own genetic molecules. It is interesting to learn that every living entity on earth has the very same genetic molecules in their chromosomes. It is simply the order and number of these genetic molecules that determines a species of life.

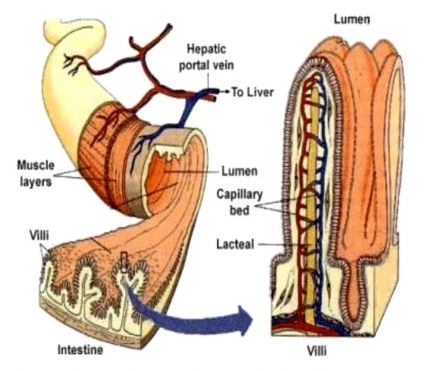

The jejunum is lined with hills and valleys called **Villi**. These hills and valleys provide a tremendous amount of surface area where the digestive process to occur. The cartoon below depicts a villus. As the intestinal muscles contract the food is squeezed into the grooved sides of the villi where enzymes perform the digestion and absorption occurs. Notice the amount of vascularity (veins and arteries) in the villi. Once absorbed the nutrients are all transported to the liver for processing. The liver is the principal biochemical factory of the body. The food moves slowly through the jejunum requiring 3-5 hours to reach the next segment of the small

The Truth About Nutrition

intestine called the **ileum.** The internal wall of the ileum continues the villi topography of the jejunum. There is no valve that separates the jejunum and the ileum. The foods pass from one segment of the small intestine to the next much like traveling from one state in the U.S. to another. The ileum is the only part of the digestive tract that absorbs vitamin B-12. It is interesting to note that B-12 is a large molecule that needs help to be absorbed. This help comes in the form of a small protein called the intrinsic factor (named before technology could analyze it). The intrinsic factor is a glycoprotein produced in the stomach that somehow does not get digested before it binds to vitamin B-12 in the distil small intestine. The B-12 intrinsic factor complex is absorbed in the ileum. Some bile is absorbed in the ileum along with other nutrients that did not get absorbed in the jejunum. The ileum ends at a muscular valve called the **ileocecal valve.**

The ileocecal valve opens usually because of the pressure exerted on the value by the food in the ileum. The opening of the valve is neurologically controlled, so abnormal pressure on that nerve can cause the valve to open prematurely allowing colon bacteria to surge into the small intestine. This can result in IBS, Irritable Bowel Syndrome, an inflammatory infection of the small intestine producing diarrhea.

When the ileocecal valve normally opens, the ileum will contract causing the food waste to pour into the **colon** (the large intestine). The food waste can remain in the colon for 20 to 30 hours. A fast transit time (12-15 hours) will only hold the food waste for a short 5 to 8 hours. The function of the colon is to prepare the food waste for disposal and to absorb much of the water from all of the digestive fluids secreted in the small intestine. Some minerals are absorbed in the colon.

The bacterial content of the colon commonly includes about 12 species, one of which is E. coli (Escherichia coli). Some of the bacterial species can be infectious to humans. The populations of most of the more infectious organisms are kept in check by waste products produced by the most common bacteria. All the bacteria in the colon produce waste products that are toxic. They can irritate the colon causing inflammation. This leads to infections further damaging the colon wall. The colon wall becomes weak causing it to form pockets called **diverticula.** These diverticular pockets can become infected. This condition is called **diverticulitis.** The condition is characterized by abdominal pain and daily, often uncontrollable diarrhea. Untreated this condition leads to colon cancer, because the reactive toxins produced by the microorganisms in the colon can cause mutations in the DNA in the colon cells. These mutations can lead to a loss of control of the cell cycle causing run-away cell division or cancer. Colon cancer is the second leading cause of cancer deaths in the U.S and the third most common form of all cancers. (CDC)

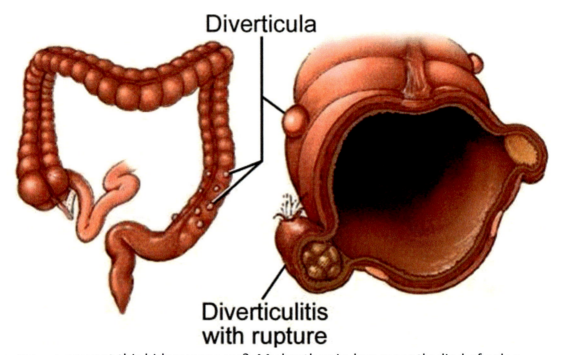

How can we prevent this hideous cancer? My brother-in-law recently died of colon cancer at 53 years of age. The answer is that this form of cancer is almost totally preventable. The main answer is **FIBER!** The average American male according to the USDA (United State Department of Agriculture) consumes 18 grams of fiber per day, whereas the average female consumes only 15 grams. These values are a far cry from the recommended 25-40 grams. Remember that fiber causes a decrease in transit time. Extended transit times allow the toxins from the colon bacteria to attack the colon walls. The bacteria in the colon can digest and metabolize dietary wastes that were useless to us, producing cancer causing toxins. I personally know many people who have a bowel movement every three days or more. Ideally you should have a remarkable bowel movement at least once a day. Twice a day would be better. If you must sit on the toilet for an extended period of time to produce a sizeable stool, you need more fiber in your diet. At a national conference on Nutrition and Preventive Medicine a doctor that was giving a research presentation was ask to describe a healthy stool. He answered that a healthy stool should be "flocculent and floating". A voluminous high fiber stool is acted upon in the colon by bacteria that produce gas. The gas bubbles cause the stool to float.

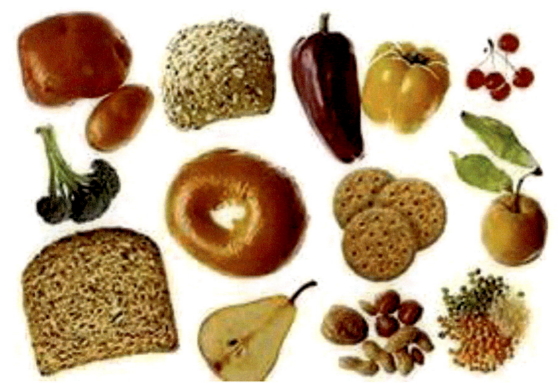

SOURCES OF FIBER – INSOLUBLE FIBER FROM NUTS, SEEDS, LEGUMES AND WHOLE GRAINS PROMOTE RAPID TRANSIT. SOLUBLE FIBER FROM FRUIT AND VEGETABLES SLOW TRANSIT.

CHAPTER 6 - METABOLISM

In the previous chapters, we have discussed the consumption of carbohydrates, lipids, and protein. We have explored how we digest each class of nutrients into small, simple molecules that we absorb into the blood stream. All the blood that receives these simple molecules goes to the liver via the portal vein. The liver is the "central warehouse of nutrients."

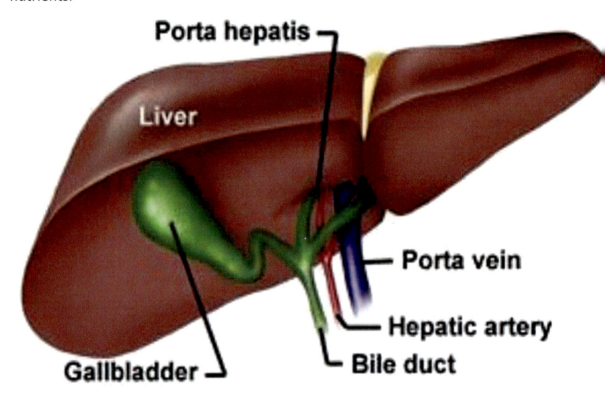

An interesting analogy can be described as: farmers grow food. They harvest the food and transport it to a farmer's market, where they distribute the food to numerous individuals. The liver is like the farmer's market. The liver is the central processing factory for all nutrients. Sugars and fats can be stored in the liver or they can be sent through the *inferior vena* cava to the heart for distribution to all the cells of the body. The liver can convert any dietary sugar into glucose. Lipids are repackaged by the liver from chylomicrons to lipoproteins. Triglycerides are mostly converted into Very Low Density Lipoproteins (VLDL). Cholesterol is synthesized into Low Density Lipoprotein (LDL) and some High-Density Lipoprotein **(HDL)**.

Amino acids can be synthesized into some proteins in the liver. The liver can convert excess non-essential amino acids into other amino acids. Once the nutrients have traveled through the liver and out to the cells of the body, the cells must decide what to do with the nutrients. The massive sum of these chemical reactions is what we call **metabolism.**

Metabolism is extremely complex. We are still learning about some of intricacies of metabolism. Some nutrients are synthesized into complex molecules to be used for cell growth, repair, and reproduction. These synthesis processes are collectively called **Anabolism.**

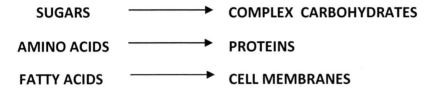

SUGARS	→	COMPLEX CARBOHYDRATES
AMINO ACIDS	→	PROTEINS
FATTY ACIDS	→	CELL MEMBRANES

All of those processes need energy, so some of the nutrients are used to produce cellular energy called **Adenosine TriPhosphate, ATP.** All living beings run on ATP, from the single celled bacteria to the very complex human being. This is the gasoline of life. These energy producing reactions are collectively called **Catabolism.**

FATTY ACIDS AND GLUCOSE ⟶ CARBON DIOXIDE + WATER + ATP

Notice that amino acids are not included as an energy source in the above equation. That is because amino acids are conserved to make protein in the body, since protein molecules are the workers in metabolism and most other tasks in the body. Do we burn some amino acid? Of course, we do. We do not always have the proper amino acid ratio necessary to make human protein, so the excess amino acids must be catabolized. The over consumption of protein lead to amino acid catabolism since we have no storage facility for protein. Observe in the equation above that fatty acids and glucose are the primary energy sources in catabolism. Fatty acids provide 9 Calories /gram and Glucose provides 4 Calories/gram. The waste molecules are carbon dioxide, which we exhale and water that leaves the body as perspiration and urine. The energy product is ATP.

Where does the energy come from in fatty acids and glucose? The answer is primarily the hydrogen atoms that are picked off of the molecules two at a time by enzymes called **dehydrogenases.** Remember that protein function because of their specific shape. For many enzymes to form their specific shape, they need what we call a **coenzyme.**

Coenzymes are either a vitamin or a mineral. In the case of dehydrogenases there are two commonly used coenzymes, vitamin B-2 (riboflavin), and vitamin B-3 (niacin). They couple together with nucleotides to form **Flavin-Adenine Dinucleotide, FAD, Flavin MonoNucleotide, FMN, Niacinamide-Adenine Dinucleotide, NAD,** and **NADP, Niacinamide-Adenine Dinucleotide Phosphate.** These coenzymes literally carry the hydrogen atoms to the mitochondria in the cell where they can be safely de-energized to make water. In a laboratory, when we take some hydrogen and mix it with oxygen, then ignite the mixture, we get a violent explosion. Obviously, we could not survive such an event occurring in our cells all over the body. The hydrogen atoms are removed from a glucose or a fatty acid molecule, then they are carried by NAD to another hydrogen carrier

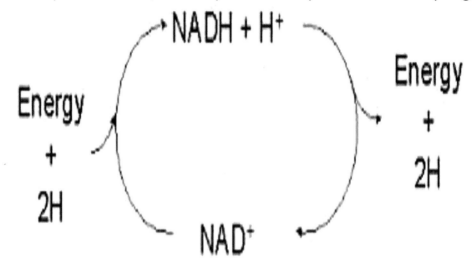

that receives the hydrogen with a slight loss of energy.

Consider the cartoon below that depicts the conversion of glucose (a 6-carbon molecule) to pyruvate (a 3 C molecule). The cartoon also depicts the conversion of pyruvate to lactate (lactic acid) which occurs in muscles when there is a lack of oxygen. The accumulation of lactic acid in the muscle causes a burning sensation, followed by pain and possible cramping of the muscle.

This metabolic pathway is called **Glycolysis** which takes place in the cytoplasm of the cells. This process is reversed when oxygen is restored to the muscle with proper circulation. Massage of the muscle and proper breathing augment this recovery. The pyruvate molecules enter the mitochondria where they are completely destroyed into CO_2 and H_2O and producing ATP

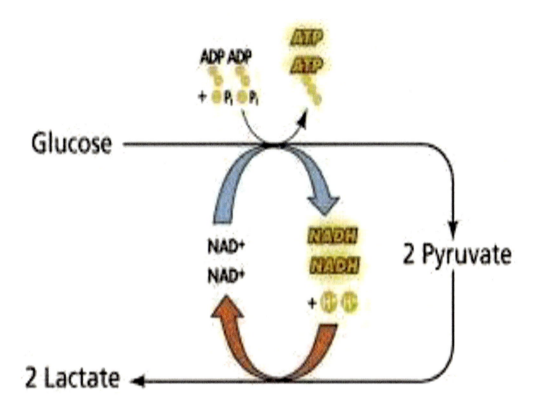

This cartoon depicts the 6-carbon glucose being converted to the 3 carbon, pyruvic acid producing ATP and hydrogens being carried by NAD.

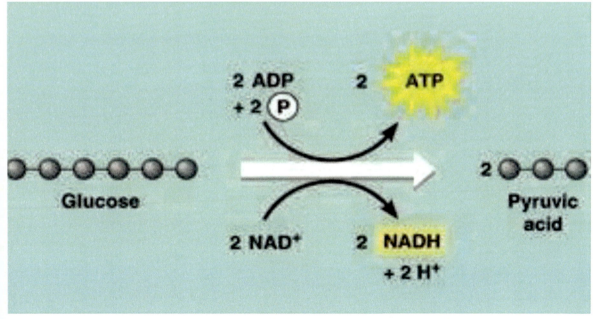

If you could make ATP in a container in your kitchen, the container would literally get ice cold as the ATP molecules sucked in the heat from the surroundings. That heat energy is stored in the chemical bonds of the phosphates.

The last phosphate bond has the most energy store in it, thus we usually see

$$ATP \longrightarrow ADP + P + E$$

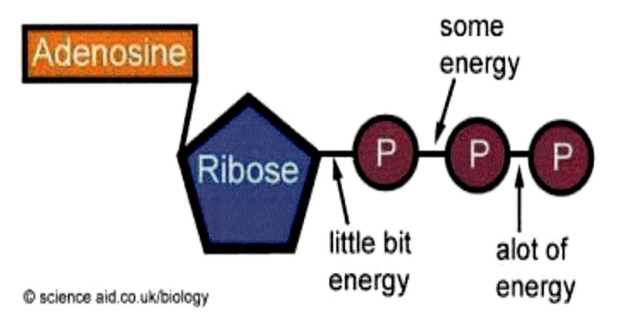

This is a constant cycle of forming ATP, losing its energy and forming ADP, then ADP receiving another high-energy phosphate reforming ATP.

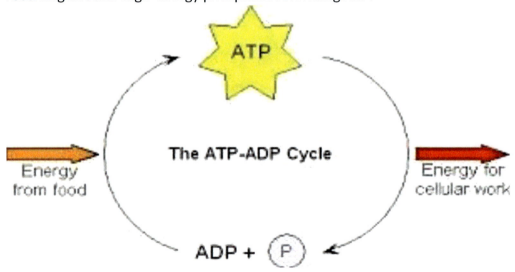

The Truth About Nutrition

What do think would happen if you did not have sufficient amounts of vitamins B-2 and B3? Clearly you could not make ATP and you would die! This is our first look at why and how important vitamins are in our nutritional regimen. This is only the beginning. The science of nutrition is a very complicated subject.

Since all of metabolism occurs in cells, it seems appropriate to look at a cell structure so that we can use the vocabulary of the cell to further our discussion of metabolism. A cell is like a city in that it has a governing center called the nucleus. This is the place that contains the genetic material we call **DNA**. The DNA is housed in highly protected structures called **chromosomes** (literally means colored bodes). We can visualize chromosomes in cells with the proper stain and a good microscope. The DNA is tightly wound around proteins so that

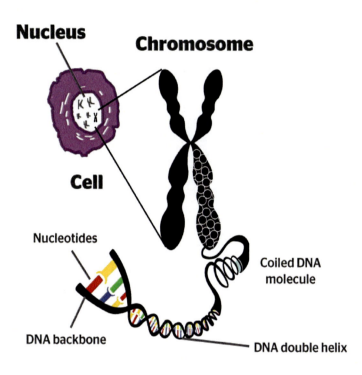

6.5 feet of DNA can be stuffed in a microscopic ball called the nucleus. The human body contains trillions of cells and over 10 billion miles of DNA, if stretched linearly end to end. A double layer of cell membrane protects the nucleus. There are structures in the membrane that can open and close to allow traffic in and out of the nucleus.

Catabolism mostly occurs in the mitochondria. The number of mitochondria in a cell varies greatly. Muscle cells for example have many mitochondria because they use so much energy contracting. Anabolism occurs in several places in the cell. Genetic material is synthesized in the nucleus. Proteins are synthesized in the Rough Endoplasmic Reticulum, RER. The rough comes from the small dots that are seen under a powerful microscope. These dots are called ribosomes that turn out to be protein factories.

Complex carbohydrates and lipids are manufactured in a region called the Smooth Endoplasmic Reticulum, SER.

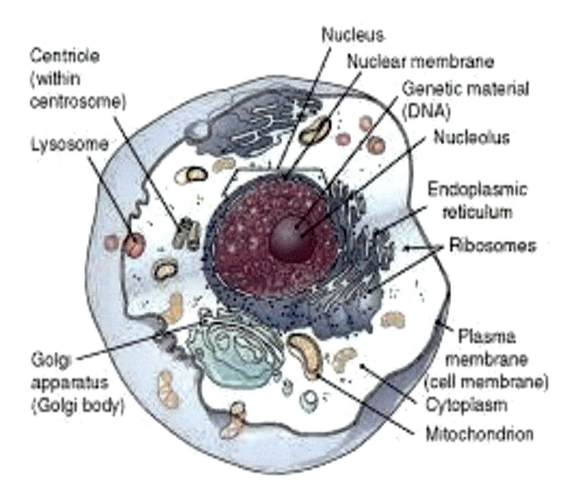

Think of catabolism as a molecular grinder for high energy food molecules. The energy is mostly in the hydrogens attached to the molecules. The mission is to convert carbon atoms to carboxyl groups, -COOH, so that enzymes (decarboxylases) can remove carbon dioxide, CO_2. The hydrogens are removed two at a time, combined with oxygen to form water, H_2O. This process releases lots of energy to be sucked up in the bonds of ATP, life's energy molecule. Every process in your body requires the energy from ATP.

Your body uses most of the consumed Calories just to live. These life processes include the beating of the heart, brain activity, breathing, kidney function, liver function, glandular function. Most people take these processes for granted, not realizing that they consume most of our energy. Collectively they are called Basal Metabolic Rate or BMR which consumes 60-70% of your total energy. The processing of food that you eat including chewing, swallowing, digesting and absorption burns 10-15% of your energy and is called the Thermal Effect of Food or TEF. So, during a 24- hour period your body will use 70-85% of the Calories you consume just to live.

Moving your body during walking, running, dancing, climbing, or any form of exercise requires the energy from ATP. Initially your muscles begin to burn glucose, but after 20-30 minutes of exercise you begin to burn fat. Aerobic exercise is any activity that raises your heart rate to what is called your Target Heart Rate. How do you determine your target heart rate? You use the following formula using 220 as the maximum heart rate and your Resting Heart Rate (pulse rate lying in bed in the morning}:
220 - Your Resting Heart Rate – Your age X 80% + Resting Heart Rate

```
Example:  220    Maximum Heart Rate
          -70    Resting Heart Rate
          - 50   Your age
          100
          X .80  80% of your maximum heart rate
          80
          + 70   Your Resting Heart Rate
          150    Your Target Heart Rate (THR)
```

This means that when you perform aerobic exercise at your 80% target heart rate you getting aerobic conditioning. Your heart and your respiratory system are both being conditioned to be more efficient. Ironically, when you are doing aerobics at your 80% THR you are only burning 40% fat after about 15 minutes. The muscles burn glucose more efficiently than fat. If you slow down to about 50% THR you burn about 55% fat. So, if your goal is to burn fat, you want to perform your aerobic exercise at a lower heart rate. Using the example above, you would lower your heart rate from 150 to 120 to burn more fat. One of the subtle benefits of aerobic exercise is that you continue to burn calories after you finish the aerobic exercise, called the "after burn". This amounts to 65 – 150 Calories depending on your weight and the intensity and duration of your exercise. The following list displays the multiple benefits of aerobic exercise:

- Increases the thermic effect of food
- Increases the production of antioxidant enzymes
- Lowers resting heart rate

- Increases the number of cellular receptor sites
- Increases muscle mass
- Decreases fat stores
- Stimulates the production of Endorphins
- Enhances the body's immune system
- Decreases the onset of degenerative diseases
- Decreases LDL and increases HDL
- Optimizes cardiopulmonary function and efficiency
- Increases the number of capillaries throughout the body
- Increases metabolic rate
- Increases the size and number of mitochondria
- Increases the body's efficiency of removing waste.

Weight lifting or Resistance Training is an anaerobic exercise, meaning that you are not increasing the efficiency of your cardiorespiratory systems. Your muscles are using the ATP stores available to them. When your muscles begin to run out of oxygen they begin converting pyruvate to lactic acid. This creates the muscle burn that can lead to muscle cramping and soreness post exercise. The principal benefit is that you Resistance Training promotes the synthesis of new muscle cells, which means that you will have more "Fat Burners" available for use.

Metabolism is a very complex phenomenon. There is no magical way to increase your metabolism. There are many people making large amounts of money selling pills that are supposed to increase your metabolism. Most of them are merely chemical stimulant that raise your heart rate so you burn more Calories. Technically, there are many hormones that help regulate metabolism. As we learn more about them, some of them will come on the market as supplements that may actually increase your metabolic rate. Some of these hormones are listed below:

METABOLIC HORMONES
- ADIPONECTIN – stimulates glucose and fat burn
- LEPTIN – reduces appetite
- GHRELIN – increase appetite
- RESISTIN – regulates lipid metabolism
- NEUROPEPTIDE Y, NPY – regulates glucose metabolism
- PANCREATIC PEPTIDE, PP – anti-obesity hormone

- ANANDAMIDE – potent hunger promoter
- ALPHA MELANOCYTE-STIMULATING HORMONE – αMSH suppresses hunger. Adiponectin and Leptin work synergistically to regulate metabolism. Ghrelin work against the synergistic pair. Adiponectin and Leptin are both protein hormones produced in fat cells. Obesity reduces the number of leptin receptor sites creating leptin resistance. As the leptin effect is diminished, the more weight is gained as fat is produced and deposited. It is a self-fulfilling prophecy. (Adapted from: Bateman, J. Supplement to Human Nutrition. Kendall/Hunt Publishing. 2000.)

ENERGY BALANCE

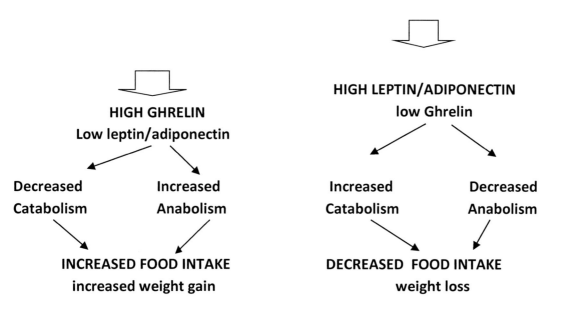

CHAPTER 7 - METABOLISM AT WORK: CARBOHYDRATES

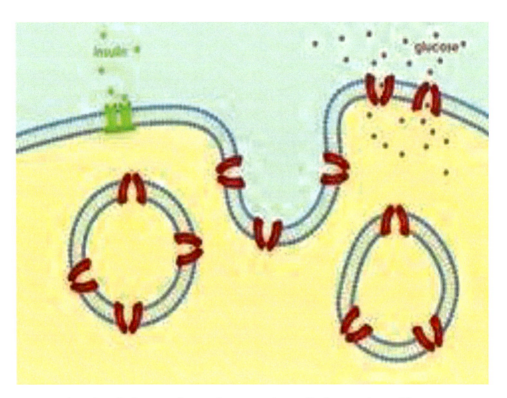

Let's trace a molecule of glucose from the mouth until absorption. There are no enzymes in the mouth, stomach or small intestine that effect glucose. Glucose simply gets mixed with saliva and other foods into a food ball. Once swallowed the glucose travels down the esophagus to the stomach where the entire food ball gets showered with gastric juice. The food ball (chyme) is squeezed into the duodenum of the small intestine where it is mixed with pancreatic juice and bile. The chyme passes into the jejunum where glucose is absorbed into the blood stream. Glucose travels in the blood to the liver where some of it may be converted to glycogen for storage. The liver can convert other sugars into glucose. The remaining amount of glucose travels out of the liver to the heart where it is pumped out through the aorta to the cells of the body. By this time the brain has detected the presence of glucose and has alerted the pancreas to release insulin. Insulin is a small protein hormone that targets insulin receptor sites in the cell membranes of the cells all over the body.

Remember that the liver, brain, and kidneys do not need insulin to absorb glucose. When insulin is received into the receptor sites it triggers the activation of the glucose transport

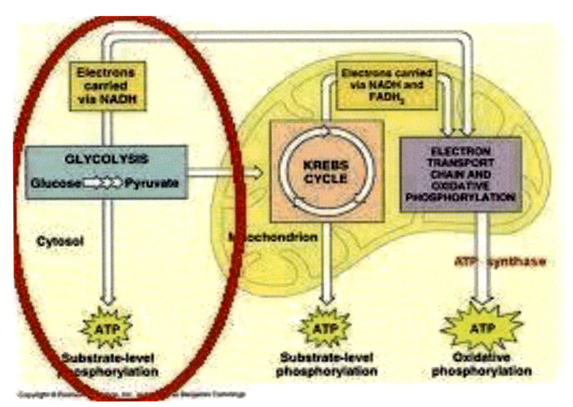

system in the cell called the *glut 4 transport system.* That system normally resides in the cytoplasm of the cell in an inactive state called a vesicle. Once activated by insulin, the vesicle joins with the cell membrane and become an active glucose transporter. Glucose enters the cells via the glut 4 ports. When blood glucose levels drop, insulin backs out of the receptors shutting down the glut 4 system. The glut 4 vesicles again take up residence in the cytoplasm in an inactive state. Have you noticed that nothing is easy in the cell?

In the cell glucose molecules are attacked by enzymes and converted from a six-carbon molecule into two three carbon molecules of *pyruvate*. Pyruvate then enters the mitochondria where it is converted into a two-carbon fragment (acetyl) that is picked up by coenzyme A, a complex containing the B vitamin, pantothenic acid (B-5). The third carbon is converted to carbon dioxide. The complex *acetyl coenzyme A* transfers the acetyl fragment into the Krebs Cycle where it joins another four-carbon molecule to form a six-carbon molecule called *citric acid*. As the citric acid and subsequent molecules encounter one enzyme after another, carbon atoms are removed as carbon dioxide as shown below. Each glucose molecule provides two pyruvates. The hydrogens are carried by either NAD+ or FAD to the **ELECTRON TRASPORT SYSTEM, ETS.** The ETS plays the game of pass the hot potato. Each time the potato is passed on, it loses some of its energy. The hypothetical hot potato is the electron from the hydrogen atom. Once the energy has been extracted from those electrons, they unceremoniously jump on an oxygen atom where two hydrogen atoms join them to form water. That escaping energy is used to form the high-energy bonds of **ATP**. One could argue that we run on burning hydrogen atoms. This is not a bad alternative to power our transportation needs.

The ETS is a set of enzymes that are sequentially located in the inner membrane of the mitochondria. Some of the enzymes contain iron. One of the hydrogen receptor molecules is called **Ubiquinone or Coenzyme Q 10**. Research has shown that as humans age, they produce less and less of the vital Coenzyme Q 10. This has become a vital supplement to help aging hearts and other muscles produce the amount of ATP necessary for a healthy life. [6]

Virtually all of the water-soluble vitamins are involved in Energy Metabolism at one time or another. Many minerals are also involved in energy metabolism. They all work together in this beautifully choreographed molecular symphony. So, what happens if you do not have adequate amount of these micronutrients? The answer is that the cells do not make enough energy to efficiently perform their function, thus you begin to be sluggish. Your energy level wains and your immune system is weakened. You become easy prey to virus and bacterial infections as well as an increased rate of aging. With

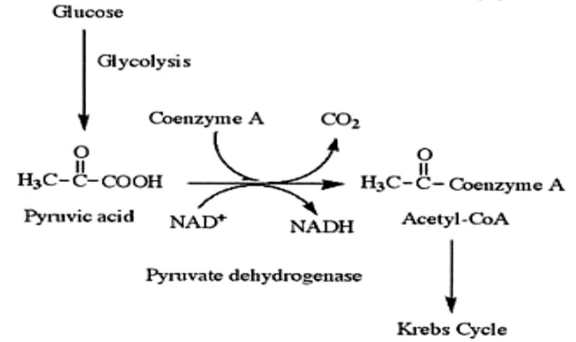

[6] Saha and Whayne. "Coenzyme Q-10 in Human Health: Supporting Evidence?" South Medical Journal. 109:17-21. January 2016.

today's technology, it is fool-hardy to not take a good multiple vitamin/mineral supplement. If you could add a can of "Engine Life" to your automobile engine that would extend its life by 100,000 miles for $12.95, would you do it? Of course, you would. We often take better care of our things than we do ourselves. What is wrong with us?

Can we get sufficient amounts of water soluble vitamins by just eating food? What is a sufficient amount? The FDA (Food and Drug Administration) sets the RDA (Recommended Dietary Allowance) values. Many professionals view these values as absolute minimums. The argument is that these minimum values do not support a human being performing at optimal levels of efficiency. In response to these views, the NAS (National Academy of Sciences) has published another set of values called the DRIs (Dietary Reference Intake). DRIs are two to several times greater than the RDAs. Some nutritional experts recommend more of a *shotgun* approach by suggesting consuming 30 – 50 % more than the DRI values. This requires a word of **CAUTION**. Excessive amounts of water soluble vitamins can overload the kidneys, making them work harder than necessary to remove the excess nutrients. This can lead to kidney diseases. You cannot live without your kidneys. The conclusion is that more is not always better. This author thinks that if we observe DRI upper limit values that we should be safe and still attain an optimal efficiency level. Observe the comparison chart below (DV = Daily Value based on aa 2000 Cal. intake):

TABLE 14 - MICRONUTRIENTS

MICRONUTRIENT	RDA	DV	DRI UL
Thiamine B-1	1.2 mg	1.5*	-
Riboflavin B-2	1.3 mg	1.7	-
Niacin B-3	16 mg	20	35
Biotin	30 mcg	300 mcg	-
Pantothenic acid B-5	5 mg	10	-
Pyridoxal B-6	1.7 mg	2	100
Folacin B-9	400 mcg	400	1000
Cyanocobalamin B-12	2.4 mcg	6	-

The Truth About Nutrition

MICRONUTRIENT	RDA	DV	DRI UL
Ascorbic acid C	90 mg	60	2000
Calcium	1200 mg	1000	2500
Magnesium	420 mg	400	350
Iron	8 mg	18	45
Zinc	11 mg	15	40
Selenium	55 ucg	70	400
Copper	900 ucg	2000	10,000
Manganese	2.3 mg	2	11
Molybdenum	45 mcg	75	2000
Sodium	2400 mg	2400	2400
Potassium	3500 mg	3500	3500
Retinal Vit A	3000 iu	5000	3000
Cholecalciferol Vit D	400 iu	400 iu	2000 iu
d-alphatocopherol E	15 mg 50 iu	9 mg 30 iu	1K mg 3333iu

*Unit of measure in the DV and DRI columns are the same as RDA. RDI values are the upper permissible values.   Vitamins A, D, E and K are Fat Soluble Vitamins. DRI UL = DRI UPPER LIMIT

The Truth About Nutrition

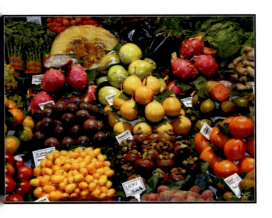
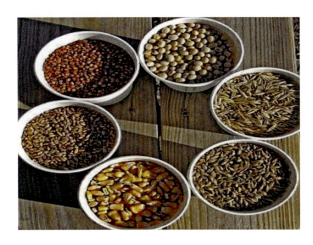

The main issue with choosing foods that provide adequate amounts of micronutrients is keeping the calories under control. Caloric Balance is Calorie In = Calories Out. Typically, animal products have a lot of Calories whereas vegetables have very few calories. Nuts, seeds, legumes, and oils are high in Calories. Most fruits and grains have a moderate number of Calories. When planning a meal, we need to think about a variety of whole grains and vegetables that we can choose. Leafy green vegetables and highly colored vegetables are always good choices, like spinach, kale, broccoli, purple cabbage, and red lettuce because they contain disease fighting chemicals. Choosing grains is often a more difficult task because food processing has given us so many tempting choices, most of which are not quality foods. There are some good cereal choices and some very good bread choices. When you observe the cereal aisle in a grocery store you will find that most of the boxes of cereal have no whole grains and high sugar contents. Food manufacturers are catering to our addictions. If you survey the bread aisle you will find that most available breads are WHITE. There are no

The Truth About Nutrition

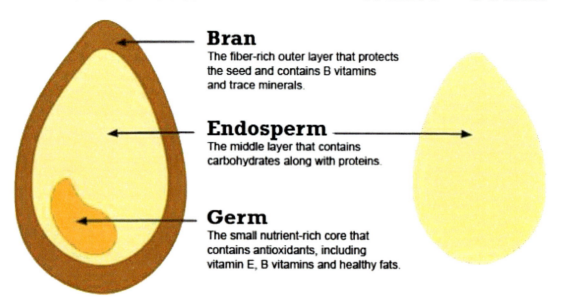

Whole Grain vs. "White" Grain

Bran — The fiber-rich outer layer that protects the seed and contains B vitamins and trace minerals.

Endosperm — The middle layer that contains carbohydrates along with proteins.

Germ — The small nutrient-rich core that contains antioxidants, including vitamin E, B vitamins and healthy fats.

white whole grains. This means that the grains have been processed. What does that look like? A whole grain has a hard covering called the bran layer. This is where most of the fiber is found. The germ is where we find most of the nutrients because it contains the embryo of the plant. The endosperm is mostly starch which provides an energy source for the growing embryo. Food processing removes the bran and the germ, leaving us with the naked starch that is often bleached to make it lily white (a symbol of purity).
What a tragedy. This process has contributed to obesity and the health decline of the modern world. Why has it taken over 100 years for intelligent people to "wake up and smell the coffee"?

When you are choosing boxed or otherwise packaged food, you must read the labels. The ingredients are listed in decreasing amounts in the food. So, if sugar is the first or second ingredient you know that you are looking at a BAD food. Food manufacturers by law add vitamins B-1, B-2, B-3, iron and folacin (B-9) to "FORTIFY" the food because all of these were removed during processing of the grain. We are still cheated out of 64% of the available micronutrients that were in the unprocessed grain. Is it any wonder that most Americans are deficient in magnesium, zinc, manganese, chromium, selenium, vitamins A, E and D along with vitamin B-6, pyridoxal. It has been wisely stated that when you are shopping for food, do most of your shopping around the perimeter of the store. This is where you will find most of the fresh foods.

Following the Mediterranean Pyramid, let's compare a couple of daily food plans to see if we can at least get RDA levels of micronutrients. We will use 1200 Calories for an average female and 2000 Calories for an average male. In this example menu, we have 3 servings of whole grains, two servings of oil, 5 servings of vegetables, one serving of fruit, 2 servings of nuts and legumes, two servings of dairy and one serving of egg.

TABLES 15 AND 16 - MEDITERRANEAN MENU FOR A FEMALE

FOOD CHOICES	AMOUNT	FOOD CHOICES	AMOUNT
Black Beans	0.5 cup	Olive Oil	2 tbsp.
Kale	1 cup	Bread mixed grain	2 slices
Parsley	1 cup	Cashews	1 oz
Quinoa	1 cup	Egg, Fried	1
Grapefruit	0.5	Tomato, raw	1 cup
Onion, raw	1	Mushrooms, cooked	0.5 cup
Coffee	1 cup	Yogurt	0.33 cup
Cottage cheese	0.5 cup	Water	8 oz

Calories = 1244   Fiber = 26

ANALYSIS

NUTRIENT	AMOUNT	RDA
Calcium	546 mg	1200 mg
Iron	14 mg	18 mg
Magnesium	390 mg	420 mg
Potassium	2497 mg	3500 mg
Sodium	742 mg	2400 mg
Zinc	8.6 mg	11 mg
Vitamin A	1293 RE	3000 RE

The Truth About Nutrition

NUTRIENT	AMOUNT	RDA
B-1	1.04 mg	1.2 mg
Vitamin E	8.4 iu	15 iu
B-2	1.51 mg	1.3 mg
B-3	10.9 mg	16 mg
B-6	1.14 mg	1.7 mg
B-9	417 mcg	400 mcg
Vitamin C	153 mg	90 mg

Analysis shows that only vitamins B2, B-9 and Vitamin C meet or exceed the RDA values. Keep in mind that these are bare minimum values and are probably not enough for a healthy individual to operate at optimal levels of efficiency. It is also important to note that a person does not need to consume optimal amounts of micronutrients every day, but should average optimal values over a week or so. There must to be a process involved in making food choices for a daily menu. Let's start with a protein choice. There are always two considerations, one is the Mediterranean Pyramid and two, the quality criteria of the nutrient class being contemplated. The pyramid shows fish, poultry, dairy or eggs as our primary choices for protein. Yes, we get some protein from grains, nuts, and legumes, but remember that none of them have all of the essential amino acids that we need to make our own proteins. We can supply all the essential amino acids by combining grains and legumes, but the efficiency is very low. The animal sources previously mentioned are the most efficient sources available. One other consideration is that the animal sources provide vitamin B-12, which is vital in the synthesis of hemoglobin and DNA synthesis. There are no commonly consumed plant sources of vitamin B-12. Americans typically love their beef and pork, but these should be consumed sparingly according to the pyramid, because of their high saturated fat content and high Calorie

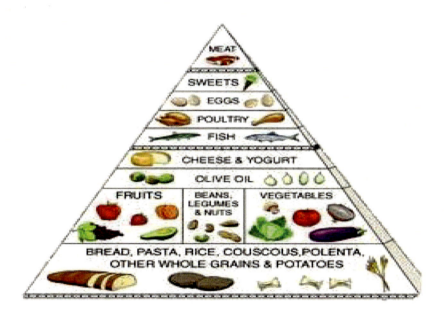

content. Sparingly means no more than once or twice per month. Seafood and poultry can be consumed weekly.

The carbohydrate nutrient class is featured in the bottom three rungs of the pyramid which include wheat, rye, barley, corn, oats, rice, millet, bulgur wheat, freekeh and quinoa (technically a seed). These grains can be served as bread, cereal, pasta, or simply by themselves. They can be included in soups or mixed with vegetables and served as a side dish. Most of the grains are good sources of insoluble fiber which decreases transit time. Observe that both menus had adequate amounts of fiber (25-40 g). Variety is the answer to provide adequate micronutrients as well as fiber. A grain choice should be a part of at least 70% of your meals each day.

TABLE 17 - SAMPLE 2000 CALORIE MENU WITH ANALYSIS

FOOD CHOICE	AMOUNT	MICRONUTRIENT	AMOUNT	RDA
Milk, skim	0.5 cup	Calcium	588 mg	1200 mg
Cereal, raisin bran	1 cup	Iron	22.5 mg	8 mg
Egg, poached	2	Magnesium	598 mg	420 mg
Onion, raw	1	Potassium	4707 mg	3500 mg
Mushroom	0.5 cup	Sodium	1782 mg	2400 mg
Coffee	2 cups	Zinc	15.7 mg	11 mg
Blue Berries	0.5 cup	Vitamin A	1817 RE	3000 RE
Salmon	4 oz	B -1	1.81 mg	1.2 mg
Walnuts	1 oz	Vitamin E	14.3 iu	15 iu
Salad, mixed	4 oz	B – 2	2.4 mg	1.3 mg
Parsley	1 cup	B - 3	25.7 mg	16 mg
Salad dressing	1 Tbsp.	B - 6	2.35 mg	1.7 mg
Peaches, fresh	1 cup	B - 9	586 mcg	400 mcg
Cashews	1 oz	Vitamin C	141 mg	90 mg
Black Beans	0.5 cup			
Quinoa	1 cup			
Kale	1 cup			
Olive oil	2 Tbsp.			
Bread multigrain	2 slices			

Calories = 2031   Fiber = 39 g

The chart above is a sample daily meal plan for a man containing about 2000 Calories. We can observe that most of the micronutrient RDAs have been met or exceeded, but far away from an optimal level when compared to DRI Upper Limit values.

Vegetables are the next source of carbohydrate. Green and highly colored vegetables typically are low in Calories, low in carbohydrate and contain many naturally protective chemicals. The exception is legumes, which are beans and peanuts. They have low glycemic index values, fiber and are rich in micronutrients. Try to choose a variety of vegetables during a weekly meal plan, for example asparagus, black beans, green beans, beets, broccoli, Brussels sprouts, cabbage, cauliflower, eggplant, Romaine lettuce, kohlrabi, mushrooms, onions, hearts of palm, parsley, peppers, peas, spinach, squash, sweet potato, tomato, water chestnuts and watercress. Ideally you should have 5-8 servings of vegetables each day. Salads are good choices to provide a variety of vegetables in one dish. You can prepare a large salad containing Romaine lettuce, spinach, kale, garbanzo beans, green pepper, onion, celery, mushrooms, and peas and store it in a plastic container for several days with a wet paper towel. You can add fresh tomato before each serving. A nice touch is to add some nuts and mandarin orange slices to the salad as you serve it. Look at the variety of food choices in just one dish. Let's look at a nutritional analysis of the proposed salad:

TABLE 18 - ANALYSIS OF PROPOSED SALAD

MICRONUTRIENT	AMOUNT	RDA
Calcium	78	1200
Iron	13.7	8 – 18
Magnesium	56	420
Potassium	495	3500
Sodium	42	2400
Zinc	1.6	11
Vitamin A	350	3000
B-1	0.4	1.2
Vitamin E	9	15
B-2	0.17	1.3
B-3	1.5	16
B-6	0.24	1.7

B-9	106	400
Vitamin C	54	90

Calories = 189   Fiber = 10 g

The nutritional analysis shows that in one dish we have satisfied 6 to 60% of the RDAs and 50% of the fiber. How can you not spend the time to prepare such nutritious foods? This salad also consists of 2 -3 servings of vegetables.

The pyramid calls for 2-3 servings of fruit per day. Fruits typically have a **low glycemic index value**. They mostly contain fructose (fruit sugar) which is absorbed slowly. Remember that low glycemic index foods stimulate a small amount of insulin, so the rate of glucose leaving the blood stream is slow. Minimum insulin levels do not elicit the conversion of glucose to fat. This is a natural weight control mechanism. There is such a wide variety of fresh fruits available for consumption, for example: apples, apricots, avocados, bananas, cherries, grapefruit, oranges, mangoes, papaya, and strawberries just to mention a few. If some fresh fruits are only available seasonally, then frozen fruits are the next best thing. One trick that you can try at home is to purchase some fresh berries during their season, wash them with detergent to remove any pesticides, rinse them thoroughly in a colander, then place ice on top of the fruit. After an hour or so, the fruit will be near freezing temperature, so remove the remaining ice and place the fruit in freezer plastic bags. Put them into the freezer immediately. This technique lowers the temperature in the fruit slowly which minimizes the formation of ice crystals. The formation of ice crystals damage the cells in the fruit causing the frozen foods to be mushy. Food processors wash the fruit, then flash freeze it in liquid nitrogen at -346° F.

The last category of carbohydrate foods are the nuts and legumes which the pyramid says 1-3 servings per day. In both sample menus and the salad, we accomplished this goal. There is a wide variety of nuts available from which to choose, for example: almonds, Brazil nuts, cashews, macadamias, pecans, and walnuts to mention a few. Legumes are beans, peas, peanuts, etc. Nuts are high in Calories and fat, but much of the fat is highly unsaturated. Beans are high in Calories and unsaturated fat, but nutrient rich.

Fat is the last Calorie Nutrient category to consider. Olive oil is the first choice for a fat. Both sample menus include some olive oil. The scientific research is very clear that monounsaturated olive oil is the best oil for a healthy, disease free life style. We need to minimize saturated fat, eliminate trans fats, maximize monounsaturated fat and optimize omega 3 fat. Another good oil to use in the preparation of food is canola oil. Canola oil is the cooking oil that has the lowest amount of saturated fat, high monounsaturated fat with both omega 3 and 6 fatty acids. The only other cooking oil that has a significant amount of omega 3 fatty acids is soybean oil. All the other common cooking oils have a disproportionate amount of omega 6 fatty acids. Remember that these omega 6 fatty acids are used to make prostaglandins in abundance which leads to disease.

A fascinating observation is that in the Mediterranean Pyramid, dairy is not considered essential. The pyramid in the sixth rung states:" Dairy or a Calcium supplement". In the old basic four food group, nutritional plan, dairy products were one the basic four food groups, suggesting that we could not survive without them. For 25 years, I have taught that cow's milk was meant for baby cows, not for humans. Mother's milk was meant for humans. When you compare the two they are very different. The first big difference is the Calories where clearly the difference is in the protein and the carbohydrate. Remember that the cow's milk protein is only 82% efficient whereas the human milk protein is 100% efficient.

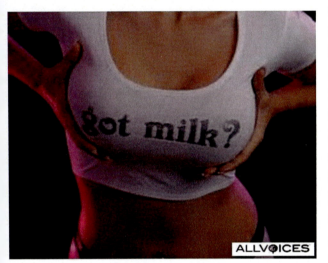

There is a slight difference in fat content, but closer observation shows that human milk fat content is more unsaturated. There is a big difference in the content of calcium, magnesium, zinc, and all the vitamins. The micronutrients that were essentially the same were intentionally omitted.

TABLE 19 - MILK COMPARISON

MILK	CAL	P	C	FIB	F	Ca	Fe	Mg	Zn	A	B1	B2	B3	B6	C
COW	150	8	11	0	8	290	.12	33	.93	76	.09	.36	.2	.1	2
HUMAN	171	2.5	17	0	11	79	.07	8	.42	178	.03	.09	.44	.03	12.3

The Truth About Nutrition

Calcium ascorbate

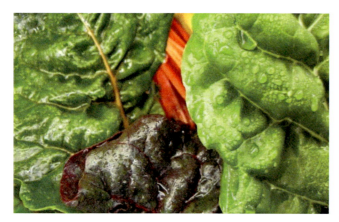

Should we consume dairy products? Of course, we should. We must remember that the fat is very saturated (70%) and we are trying to minimize saturated fat. There are very good fat free or low fat dairy product choices of which we should avail ourselves. 48% of the calories in whole milk come from fat whereas only 4% of the calories in skim milk come from fat. The biggest fallacy is that we must have dairy to get adequate calcium. The pyramid states that we can take a calcium supplement. Most calcium supplements are composed of **calcium carbonate**, which is limestone. We do not absorb this supplement very well. It is not soluble in water.

Many plant foods have a higher calcium nutrient density than milk. For example, 48 Calories of collard greens have the same amount of calcium as 96 Calories of skim milk, so collard greens have twice the nutrient density. Chinese cabbage, watercress, beet greens, parsley, rhubarb, spinach, and endive all have higher nutrient densities with respect to calcium. The calcium content of many plant foods is not as available for absorption as it is in milk. This is because much of the calcium in plants is bound to fiber from which our digestive tract has trouble liberating. Taking a vitamin C at the time you consume these plant sources of calcium can increase the calcium absorption.

Fiber intake is another consideration when planning your carbohydrate choices. Most protein and fat choices do not have appreciable amounts of fiber. Consider the fiber chart below:

TABLE 20 - FIBER CONTENT OF VARIOUS FOODS

FOOD (100 g)	ENERGY (Cal)	CARBO (g)	FAT (g)	FIBER (g)	ND$_{FIBER}$ x 100
Apples	59	15	0.5	2.8	5
Avocado	112	8.9	8.9	5.3	5
Blackberries	52	12.5	0.7	5.6	10
Figs, dried	255	65	1	9.5	4
Prunes	107	28	0.4	6.5	6
Raspberries	49	11.4	0.8	6.5	13
Mango	65	17	0.5	2	3
Bread, multigrain	250	46	4	7.7	3
Barley	123	28	0.6	3.8	3
Cereal, Bran	258	74	3.2	32	13
Cereal, Fiber one	200	83	3	47	23
Granola	451	65	17.7	6	1
Quinoa	120	4.3	2	3	3
Rice, Brown	111	23	1	2	2
Almonds	589	20	52	10.6	2
Artichoke	45	9	0.6	4.8	11
Black Beans	132	23	.23	8.2	6

The Truth About Nutrition

Broccoli	28	5	0.6	2.8	10
Sundried Tomato	257	56	3.7	13	5

The ND, Nutrient Density with respect to Fiber were all decimal numbers, so they were multiplied by 100 to establish a whole number comparison. Observe that the fruits, vegetables, and high fiber grains provide the highest fiber content. Recall that the goal is to get 25-40 g of fiber per day. Adequate fiber intake is our number one protector against the epidemic disease of cancer of the colon.

When preparing fruits and vegetables for eating, always wash them in a mild detergent and thoroughly rinse. This will remove much of the fat-soluble pesticides on the surfaces of the produce. As you are washing, cut away any spots that are brown or black because these spots contain oxidized substances that are toxic and may be carcinogenic.

CHAPTER 8 - METABOLISM AT WORK: LIPIDS

Choosing fats for your diet is challenging. There are many sources of fat to choose from including animal meat fats, egg fat, grain fat, vegetable fat and fat from nuts and seeds. It turns out that the fat from these various sources are not equal. Research has taught us that unsaturated fat is much better for our health than saturated fat. Let's compare some animal fats in the following table:

TABLE 21 - ANIMAL FAT COMPOSITION

FOOD	SAT FAT	18:0	16:0	14:0	UNSAT	MONO	16:1	18:2 Ω-6	18:3 Ω-3
BUTTER	54%	11	31%	12%	32 %	24 %	4 %	3 %	1 %
EGG	33 %				61 %	41 %		20 %	
LARD	38-43%	12-14%	25-28%	1%	56-62%	47-50%	3 %	10 %	0
TALLOW	43 %	14 %	26 %	3 %	54 %	47 %	3 %	3 %	1 %
SUET	52 %	31%	17 %	4 %	35 %	32 %	0	3 %	0

Curiously, butter has the highest saturated fat content in the list. Lard (Pig fat) has the highest unsaturated fat and the highest monounsaturated fat content. Tallow (rendered beef fat) has the second highest monounsaturated fat content. Suet (raw beef fat) has the second highest saturated fat content.

Research suggests that we should limit saturated fat to no more than 10% of our total fat intake. A daily menu of 2000 Calories should contain no more that 30% fat or 600 Calories of fat. 10% of that would be 60 Calories. An egg contains 5.9 grams of fat with 33% of it being saturated. This would be approximately 2 grams of saturated fat. Two eggs would provide 4 grams of saturated fat or 36 Calories, below the 60 Calorie maximum.

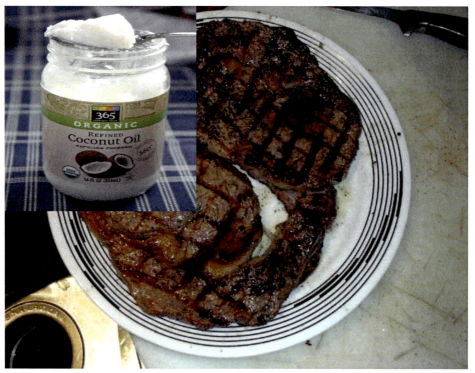

A modest serving of sirloin steak is 3 ounces or 84 grams, which would contain 12 grams of fat and 5 grams or 45 Calories of saturated fat. If you ate both in the same day you would consume 81 Calories of saturated fat, considerable over the hypothetical 60 Calorie limit. You can see that lower fat choices like chicken or fish would be much wiser. Plant choices of fat are mostly low in saturated fat except for Palm oil and Coconut oil. Nuts and seeds are usually high in fat, but not saturated fat. For example, one ounce of corn oil has 7 grams of saturated fat, while peanut oil has 5.3 grams of saturated fat in one ounce. In comparison, one ounce of coconut oil has 27 grams of saturated fat. It certainly does not make any sense to choose coconut oil as nutritional component of one's diet, since 90% of the oil is saturated fat. Observations of the chart on the next page shows that the fat choices that is the highest in monounsaturated fatty acids (MUFA's) are olive oil, canola oil and almond oil. The highest sources of polyunsaturated fatty acids are flaxseed oil, safflower oil and walnut oil. The highest sources of omega 3 (n-3) fatty acids are flaxseed oil, canola oil and walnut oil. Since we need monounsaturated fatty acids and omega 3 polyunsaturated fatty acids (PUFA's), a combination of these sources is highly advisable.

TABLE 22 - FAT CONTENT OF PLANT FOODS

SOURCE	SATURATED	MONOUSF	PUFA	18:2 n-6	18:3 n-3
COCONUT	90	9	0.5	0.5	0
CORN	25	27	48	48	0
FLAXSEED	10	22	68	21	47
OLIVE	14	78	7	7	0
SOYBEAN	14	29	57	49	8
SUNFLOWER	9	32	59	59	0
PEANUT	19	51	22	22	0
SAFFLOWER	7	17	76	76	0
CANOLA	10	59	31	19	12
ALMOND	8	74	19.4	19.3	0.1
WALNUT	9.5	13.8	72	58.4	13.9

Lipids include fats, oils, phospholipids, and cholesterol. Fats, oils, and phospholipids contain fatty acids that can be catabolized for energy. They provide 9 Calories per gram, the highest calorie content of any food. In contrast, cholesterol cannot be catabolized for energy. It is a molecule for which we have no enzymes that can break it apart. So, we must get rid of it as is. This is difficult because cholesterol is very incompatible with water. Phospholipids are partially soluble in water. If we surround cholesterol molecules with phospholipids, we can sneak them through our water based system. We call these complexes **chylomicrons.** The destination of any nutrient is the liver. The liver is our chemical factory that can process almost anything. If the liver cannot process a substance, then it can store it. We all have toxic chemicals stored in the liver.

Research has taught us that saturated fats and excess cholesterol can lead to fatty deposits on the arteries called **atherosclerosis.** Atherosclerosis leads to CHD, coronary heart disease and eventually heart attack. What is the etiology (medical cause) of CHD?

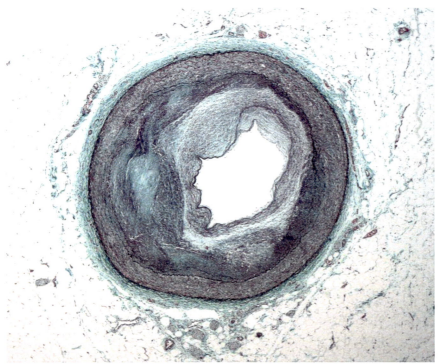

This is a little complex, so hang in there. It all starts with an unfortunate genetic inheritance of genes that causes you to mishandle fats (dyslipidemia). The dietary consumption of fats can lead to high triglycerides and high cholesterol in the blood (hyperlipidemia) and (hypercholesterolemia).

CROSS SECTION OF A DISEASED ARTERY SHOWING ATHEROSCLEROSIS AND PLAQUE

The liver packages dietary triglycerides mostly as **VLDL**, Very Low Density Lipoprotein containing ~ 10% cholesterol, while most dietary cholesterol is packaged as **LDL**, Low Density Lipoprotein, sending them to through the blood stream to the cells of the body. During transit to the LDL receptor sites in the membranes of the cells, these lipid aggregates encounter oxygen and various free radicals which attack these complexes causing oxidation. Oxidized lipoproteins are attracted to the surface of arteries where they form a sticky deposit called plaque. These oxidized lipoproteins are cytotoxic (poisonous to cells) triggering the development of sick cells causing an immune response. Chemical signals requesting help are sent via the blood stream which alerts white blood cells called neutrophils. Neutrophils proliferate in a lipid rich environment. The neutrophils enter the sick cells producing what is called an atheroma.

Large hungry white blood cells called macrophages (large eating cells) are recruited to clean up the mess. The macrophages enter the sick cells and proceed to gorge themselves with oxidized lipoproteins, oxidized cholesterol, and oxidized phospholipids. These oxidized lipids trigger the cells death program (apoptosis) causing these sick cells to die becoming "foam cells". These dead cells enlarge the atheroma attracting more oxidized cholesterol and other oxidized lipids. Sticky blood cells called platelets begin to stick to the atheroma attracting red blood cells forming a blood clot. This plugs the lumen (opening) of the artery stopping the blood flow to that tissue, resulting in the death of that tissue. If that tissue is the heart, it is called a heart attack. Choosing the wrong sources of fat can lead to dire consequences. Choose wisely my friends.

Let's explore the metabolism of lipids. As previously discussed, lipids are absorbed as complexes called chylomicrons. Shorter chain fatty acids (12 carbons or less) can be absorbed attached to small protein molecules called albumins for transport to the cells of the liver. The liver repackages the fats as the lipoprotein, VLDL. The VLDL's transport the fats to the cells of the body, particularly adipose cells. Elevated insulin levels promote excess glucose to be synthesized into fatty acids. This process requires the coenzyme NADP+ (Niacinamide Adenine Dinucleotide Phosphate that contains niacin). The newly synthesized fatty acids are shuttled to the adipose cells where they are stored as triglycerides for future use. This can lead to obesity. Remember that low glycemic index

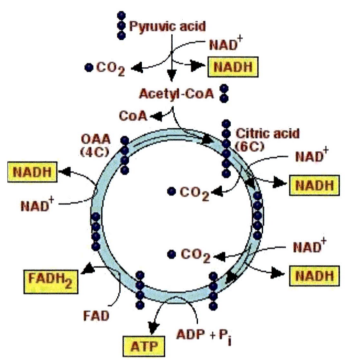

carbohydrates promote elevated levels of insulin which in turn promotes fatty acid synthesis leading to increased obesity. Remember that we only synthesize saturated fatty acids that are typically stored as long chain fatty acids (C-16 and C18). This makes them more difficult to recirculate. When saturated fatty acids are excessively used to make cell membranes, the membranes become more rigid leading to the malfunction of the cell.

Elevated levels of epinephrine (adrenaline) and glucagon stimulate the beta oxidation cycle (fatty acid cycle) which converts fatty acids into short, two carbon fragments called acetyl groups. All fatty acid fragments are carried by coenzyme A that contains pantothenic acid (vitamin B-5). The fatty acid cycle also requires the coenzymes FAD AND NAD+ which contain riboflavin (vitamin B-2) and niacin (vitamin B-3) respectfully. Acetyl groups attached to coenzyme A are burned in the Krebs cycle for energy. The fatty acid cycle and the Krebs cycle are both contained in the mitochondria of the cells, the only place this occurs.

When we use fat or carbohydrate for energy, the acetyl groups that result from the partial breakdown must pass through the Krebs cycle. The CO_2 that is removed from the acetyl groups passes through the blood stream to the lungs, where it is exhaled. The hydrogens that are removed are transported by NAD+ and FAD to the ETS, Electron Transport System, where their energy is slowly removed as they are passed from one receiver molecule after another. The ETS contains iron and copper containing protein complexes as well as riboflavin and coenzyme Q_{10}. The Krebs cycle does not run backward like the fatty acid cycle, so we cannot convert fat into sugars. The only way we can make sugar is through gluconeogenesis using amino acids as the precursor.

The Electron Transport System is pictured below. This is found in the mitochondria and is a mechanism for methodically removing energy from liberated hydrogens. Their eventual fate is to join oxygen to form water.

Metallo Flavoprotein

AH_2 — Co enzyme NAD^+ — Fe Flavin-H_2 — Co enzyme Q — $2H^*$ — $2Fe^{3+}$ — $2H^*$ — ½ O_2

A — NADH+H^* — Fe-Flavin — Q-H_2 — Cytochromes — $2Fe^{2+}$ — H_2O

Dehydrogenase Protein

We can observe the coenzymes NAD+, FMN and Coenzyme Q in the front end of the ETS. The electrons from the hydrogens are passed on to iron, Fe, and finally to a copper, Cu, containing protein before the worn-out electrons are passed to oxygens. Now the negatively charged oxygens attract the awaiting H^+ ions to form water. When two H^+ ions join an O_2 molecule they can for hydrogen peroxide, a cytotoxic molecule. Evolution has provided two protective enzyme systems to dispose of hydrogen peroxide. One of these is called Catalase that contains Fe, iron, as a coenzyme and Glutathione Peroxidase that contains Se, Selenium, as the coenzyme. Catalase is prolific in red blood cells. If you have ever put peroxide on a cut, you have probably observed the massive amount of bubbles that result. Catalase decomposes several million molecules of hydrogen peroxide per second.

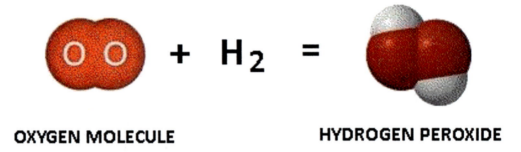

The formation of hydrogen peroxide can lead to the production of OH (hydroxyl) free radicals, the most reactive of free radicals. Remember a free radical is a molecular species with an unpaired electron. Free radicals react with any molecule as soon as possible to pair their electrons. Cell membranes, functioning proteins, and DNA molecules, etc. can be damaged or destroyed. This type of damage can lead to premature cell death. It can also lead to cancer. Another dangerous free radical is the O_2^-, called superoxide. Evolution has provided us with an enzyme that rapidly destroys superoxide. This enzyme is called SOD, Super Oxide Dismutase. The cytoplasm of the cell has a version of this enzyme that uses zinc and copper as coenzymes. Mitochondria have their own version of SOD that contains zinc and manganese as coenzymes.

Oxidation is defined as the loss of electrons. It is nature's way of getting rid of unwanted molecules. Oxidation can destroy good molecules like protein and DNA. A delicate balance must be maintained.

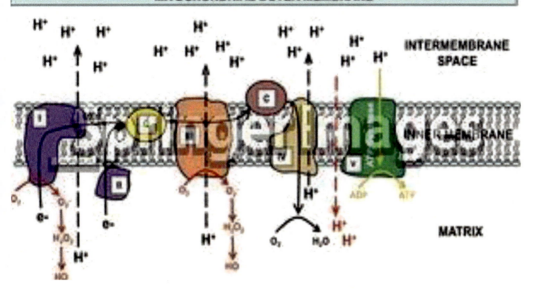

CHAPTER 9 - METABOLISM AT WORK: PROTEINS

Choosing proteins in your diet is most important. Proteins are composed of amino acids, eight or nine of which are essential (cannot be synthesized in the body). Animal proteins are the only ones that contain all the essential amino acids, but combining specific plant proteins can provide all the essential amino acids (see the protein chapter). Protein should comprise about 20% of your Calorie consumption. Some non-essential amino acids are used to synthesize the nitrogen bases that are used to build molecules of RNA and DNA. It is interesting to note that every organism that has been studied performs these syntheses in exactly the same way. Is this coincidence?

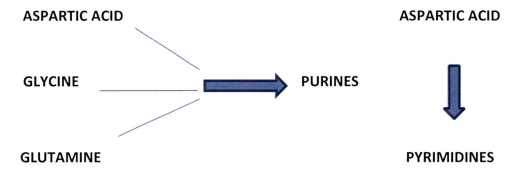

The **purines** used in nucleic acids are **ADENINE** and **GUANINE**. The **pyrimidines** used in nucleic acids are **CYTOSINE** and **THYMINE** in DNA, **CYTOSINE** and **URACIL** in RNA.

There is a sizeable need for micronutrients in the synthesis and utilization of protein. Vitamin B-6 is vital in the transport of amino acids. This is a vitamin that is difficult to obtain.

The Truth About Nutrition

TABLE 23 - SOURCES OF B-6, B-9 AND B-12

Sources B-6 (mg/oz)		Sources of Folate, B-9 ug/100g		Sources of B-12 ug/100g	
Sunflower seeds	0.38	Black-eyes peas	208	Clams	98.9
Pistachio nuts	1.12	Lentils	181	Beef liver	83.1
Tuna	0.28	Spinach	194	Salmon	15.4
Turkey/chicken White	0.23	Asparagus	149	Crab	11.5
Pork, lean	0.23	Romaine	136	Beef	6.0
		Broccoli	108	Swiss cheese	3.34
		Avocado	81	Eggs	1.95

The synthesis or anabolism of protein is a genetically controlled process. Gene mutations can result in the synthesis of aberrant protein molecules. Since protein molecules are functional molecules, an aberrant protein could cause a normal process to be altered to cause disease. Protein synthesis is dictated by DNA and directed by messenger RNA (mRNA). The amino acid sequence (the order of amino acids in the protein chain) follows the genetic code displayed by mRNA. Most DNA and energy (ATP) reactions must have, Mg, magnesium present. Vitamins B-9 and B-12 are essential in the synthesis of DNA, RNA, and protein. The minerals Zinc (Zn) and Iron (Fe) and the "B vitamin" Biotin are essential in the synthesis and utilization of protein.

Amino acids are different than carbohydrates and fats in that they contain nitrogen as amino groups ($-NH_2$) and they cannot be stored. These amino groups must be removed from excess amino acids by enzymes called **deaminases or transaminases**. The liberated amino groups are combined with carbon dioxide to make a waste molecule called **urea,** in the urea cycle in the liver and kidneys. Nitrogen wastes are toxic, making it essential the they be removed quickly. Fortunately, we have organs called kidneys that remove urea from the blood stream allowing us to get rid of the waste as urine. Problems with your

DEAMINATION OF GLUTAMATE

$$\text{Glutamate} + H_2O \;\underset{\text{glutamate dehydrogenase}}{\overset{NAD^+ \longrightarrow NADH + H^+}{\rightleftharpoons}}\; \text{α-ketoglutarate} + NH_4^+$$

kidneys, bladder or urethra (the tube from the bladder to outside the body) can cause urine retention. Urea concentrations in the blood increase to the point of being toxic, which is known as uremic poisoning, a potentially fatal condition. After deamination, the remaining part of the amino acid molecule is metabolized like a molecule of carbohydrate. It can be methodically altered into acetyl groups that enter the Krebs Cycle where they can be catabolized or synthesized into a sugar molecule (gluconeogenesis). Gluconeogenesis is a process that is implemented when the intake of carbohydrate is restricted. It also can occur during fasting. Excess amino acids can also be used to make fat that can be stored. Ultimately this is a waste of valuable amino acids since they are uniquely made into vital proteins and nucleic acids, the main functional molecules in the cell. Observing the protein efficiency chart in the protein chapter illustrates that low efficiency protein sources lead to an excess of waste amino acids that must be catabolized.

Nitrogen balance is a concept that is vital to homeostasis (biological equilibrium). Since there are always waste amounts of amino acids because none of our sources of dietary protein are 100% efficient (see protein chapter), the excess amino acids must be destroyed. This results in a nitrogen loss. The consumption of protein represents a nitrogen gain. Ideally if you are in a state of homeostasis: **Nitrogen In** should equal **Nitrogen Out**. Since most of the dietary protein that we consume is used to build and maintain muscle tissue, a state of **Nitrogen In > Nitrogen Out** can allow you to build increased amounts of muscle protein. The reverse produces muscle wasting and increased weakness.

This is a photograph of a child that has been deprived of protein. He is showing a total lack of skeletal muscle. He is virtually skin and bones. His little abdomen is swollen due to fluid edema and an enlarged liver. Since hair is made of protein, this child does not have any. The body will not allow the use of protein to make any non-essential structures. This state of starvation is called Kwashiorkor Disease. Most of the pictures showing this disease are of children since they seldom live to become teenagers or adults.

Contrast this to the picture below showing a person who has had adequate nutrition and has exercised extensively. To maintain this state of fitness, one must continue to eat adequate amounts of high quality food including high efficiency

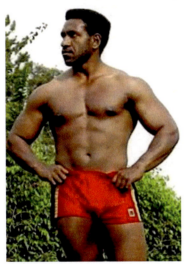

protein sources like eggs, seafood, and dairy products. They must also continue to exercise all the muscles in the body. The consumption of eggs used to be discouraged because of the content of cholesterol. Research has shown that the cholesterol in the egg does not raise the blood levels of cholesterol. So, the consumption of egg whites is no long necessary. Analysis shows that the protein content of an egg is 55% in the white and 45% in the yolk. Analysis also shows the 75-90% of the micronutrients are in the yolk of the egg and not in the white. Egg is the most efficient source of protein you can eat at 94% incorporation into human protein. Just in case you are wondering if our genetics are closely related to the chicken, let me allay your fears; we are not closely related genetically or any other way. Research has shown that there is 60% homology (gene similarity in structure and function) between chickens and humans. Of the 60%, 75% of the chicken genes were identical to the human version. Rodents display a larger identical homology at 88%, whereas Chimpanzees have a 99% identical homology. (NIH news release. "Researchers Compare Chicken and Human Genomes." <u>National Human Genome Research Institute.</u> December 8, 2004.

The Truth About Nutrition

The catabolism of purines produces a different nitrogen waste call **uric acid.** When we lose the ability to efficiently rid the body of uric acid, it can accumulate in joints causing a disease called **gout.** Gout is a genetically based disease that is turned on by a diet containing organ meats, red meat, and shell fish. Alcohol and High Glycemic Index carbohydrates stimulate the onset.

CHAPTER 10 - NUTRITIONAL SUPPLEMENTS

Why do we need nutritional supplements? There are several reasons for this need. As previously discussed in this book, most people eat a diet that does not provide optimal amounts of micronutrients. This leads to deficiencies that compromise your immune system making you susceptible to degenerative disease. In a perfect world, we would have a food intake monitoring computer that would detect the exact amounts of micronutrients that we are consuming daily. The computer would tell us the exact amounts of supplement we need to take to optimize out nutritional status. Well, guess what? We do not have such technology so we take more of a shotgun approach to supplementation. We take optimal levels of micronutrients to assure that we are consuming enough.

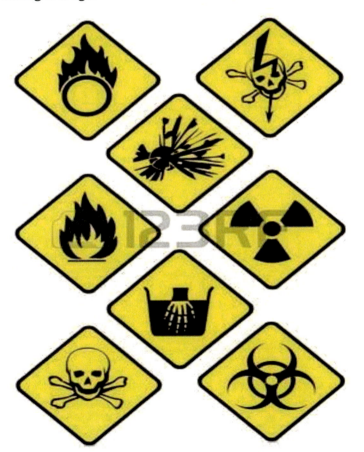

The second reason that we should take supplements is that we live in an anthropogenic (man-made) polluted world. There are toxins in the air, the water, our food, and the surroundings that we live in. New carpets outgas organic compounds into the air. Fresh paint outgases organic molecules into the air. The high-tech world we live in dictates that the pollution will continue for a long time. Supplements that bolster our immune system can help us deal with these pollutants. Most of the toxins that enter our bodies wind up in the liver where they can be stored or destroyed by the **Cytochrome P-450** enzyme system (a cellular enzyme system with powerful oxidizing capability). Our fat stores all over the body contain stored amounts of pesticides like DDT. Supplements can augment the body's natural mechanisms that deal with the toxic effects of pollutants.

A third reason for using supplements is that research continues to prove that various components of natural products can have a tremendously beneficial effect in the constant battle to thwart the
devastating effects of degenerative disease. For example, there is a mountain of evidence that there are many supplements that can help prevent cancer. We will explore some of these supplements.

There are many supplements that a person can take, some of which are rather expensive. You could easily take $10-$50 of supplements each day. The bottom line is that you need to assess what your budget can afford and then assess the most effective supplemental regime for you. In the pages that follow we will present arguments and scientific evidence for taking some supplements. No attempt will be made to include all the supplements that are available.

What constitutes a good supplement? Here are the criteria:

1. The supplement should be made by a reputable company. Research has proven that many of the over-the-counter supplements that are sold in retail stores do not have the contents that they claim to contain. (Cohen, P. "American Roulette-Contaminated Dietary Supplements." New England Journal of Medicine. 361: 1523-1525. October 15, 2009.)

2. The supplement should be in a chemical form that is readily absorbed. Most mineral supplements are in the inorganic form, like magnesium oxide. Magnesium is absorbed in the small intestine where inorganic magnesium combines with hydroxide ions and phosphate ions to form insoluble compounds. They wind up in the stool.

3. The company that manufactures the supplement should have one or two independent laboratories perform a quantitative analysis on their products to confirm their contents. This information should be readily available to the consumer. Life Extension supplements
are independently tested by two certified testing laboratories and issued a Certificate of Analysis which is available to all customers upon request. (Life Extension 2017 Directory. 10-13. November 2016.).

A good **multivitamin/mineral supplement** is this author's **number one** recommendation. The Centrum silver vitamin supplement contains the RDA levels of vitamins and minerals. For example: look at Vitamin D3. The Centrum has 500 IU whereas the **Life Extension (LE) two-per-day vitamin** has 2000 IU which is much more in accord with current recommendation in the medical literature. The person taking the centrum would have to take a vitamin D-3 supplement to achieve recommended levels – another pill, another dollar. Many researchers are recommending even higher levels of vitamin D3, around 5000 IU. Calcium, magnesium, and potassium levels in the LE multivitamin are considerably less than the optimal recommendation.

VITAMIN/MINERAL SUPPLEMENTS COMPARISON

NUTRIENT	3 SPECTRA SR.	CENTRUM 1	TWO A DAY
Vitamin A	9500 iu	2500 iu	**5000 iu**
Vitamin C	300 mg	60 mg	**500 mg**
Vitamin D-3	200 iu	500 iu	**2000 iu**
Vitamin E	200 iu	50 iu	**100 iu**
Vitamin K-1	2.5 mg	30 mcg	**0**
Thiamin B-1	25 mg	1.5 mg	**75 mg**
Riboflavin B-2	25 mg	1.7 mg	**50 mg**
Niacin B-3	25 mg	20 mg	**50 mg**
Pyridoxiine B-6	25 mg	3 mg	**75 mg**
Folacin B-9	200 mcg	400 mcg	**400 mcg**
Methylcobalamin B12	25 mcg	25 mcg	**300 mcg**
Biotin	150 mcg	30 mcg	**300 mcg**
Pantothenic Acid B-5	25 mg	10 mg	**100 mg**
Calcium	300 mg	200 mg	**25 mg**
Iodine	35 mcg	150 mcg	**150 mcg**
Magnesium	150 mg	50 mg	**100 mg**
Zinc	10 mg	11 mg	**30 mg**
Selenium	25 mcg	55 mcg	**200 mcg**
Copper	25 mcg	0.5 mg	**0**
Manganese	2.5 mg	2.3 mg	**2 mg**
Chromium	25 mcg	45 mcg	**200 mcg**
Molybdenum	25 mcg	45 mcg	**100 mcg**

The Truth About Nutrition

ım	25 mg	80 mg	**25 mg**
	0.5 mg	150 mcg	**300 mg**
Silicon	3 mg	2 mg	0
Vanadium	10 mcg	10 mcg	0
NUTRIENT	**3 SPECTRA SR.**	**CENTRUM 1**	**TWO A DAY**
Choline	50 mg	0	**20 mg**
Inositol	25 mg	0	**50 mg**
PABA	25 mg	0	0
L-cysteine	25 mg	0	0
Glutamic Acid	25 mg	0	0
dl Methionine	25 mg	0	0
L Aspartic Acid	50 mg	0	0
Phosphatidylserine	12.5 mg	0	0
Octacosanol	500 mcg	0	0
Soy lecithin	50 mg	0	0
Gammalinolenic acid	2.5 mg	0	0
Alpha Lipoic acid	15 mg	0	**25 mg**
Coenzyme Q-10	5 mg	0	0
Lutein	0.250 mg	0	**5 mg**
Lycopene	0.3 mg	0	**1 mg**
Mixed Tocopherols	0	0	**20 mg**
Niacinamide riboside	0	0	**1 mg**

When you take a multivitamin supplement, your urine may become bright yellow. This indicates that some of the vitamin B 2 (Riboflavin) has reached the kidneys and has been removed from the blood stream. This is not a problem, because the "B" vitamins are water soluble, non-toxic in these amounts and are not stored in the body. Most of the micronutrients are absorbed in the small intestine which has a basic environment, pH of 8.

The second recommendation is a **Magnesium supplement**. Most Americans (70-80%) are deficient in magnesium. There are over 6,000 research journal articles on magnesium deficiencies. It is not readily available in the average diet. Magnesium is the central ion in chlorophyll, so anything green is going to have magnesium. Nut and seeds are going to be rich in many nutrients because they are the reproductive structures of the plant. Plants surround their baby plants with necessary nutrients so they can have a good start in life.

The problem is that these sources are also high in Calories. You get more bang for your buck by eating green things. For example, a serving of spinach has only 14 Calories and supplies 44 mg of magnesium, whereas peanuts have 216 mg of magnesium but also have 223 Calories (about one and half cups). Magnesium is used as a coenzyme in over 300 biochemical reactions in the cells. As stated previously, Magnesium is required for all energy reactions in the cell, so a deficiency means you will be limited in your production and utilization of ATP. The result is low personal energy level. It is well documented in the medical literature that magnesium deficiencies promote heart disease and diabetes. (Greenfield, S. "The National Magnesium Crisis." Life Extension. 22:45-51. December 2016.)

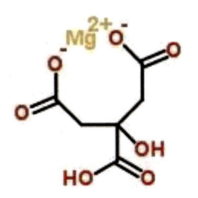

Magnesium is difficult to absorb because it forms insoluble solids in a basic medium. Many magnesium supplements contain MgO, magnesium oxide, which has a minimal bioavailability because of its low solubility in water and even less in a basic environment. A chelated (from chela = claw) form (Mg wrapped with an organic molecule) has a much higher bioavailability and therefore a greater absorption. Research at the National Institutes of Health showed that magnesium citrate was 36 times better absorbed compared to magnesium oxide. We recommend Magnesium citrate or Magnesium ascorbate.

The third recommendation is a **Calcium supplement**. If you consume dairy products frequently you probably get at least the RDA (1000 mg) of calcium. If you do not consume a lot of dairy products, then you need to eat a lot of green vegetables like Chinese cabbage, collard greens, spinach, beet greens and parsley. For example, a serving of cooked collard greens provides 35 Calories with 218 mg of calcium. A serving of low fat yogurt has 127 Calories and provides 452 mg of calcium. Like magnesium, calcium is hard to absorb unless taken in the chelate form, calcium citrate or calcium ascorbate. Vitamin D. facilitates calcium absorption

The fourth recommendation is Omega 3 (Fish oil) supplements. Nearly 21,000 research papers are currently published in the medical literature on omega 3 fatty acids. They are also known as Marine lipids. They include two long chain polyunsaturated fatty acids that can be immediately use in our bodies to produce healthy prostaglandins. These fatty acids are abbreviated as EPA, eicosapentaenoic acid, 20:5 n-3 (20 Carbons, 5 double bonds, the first one on the third carbon from the end of the molecule) and DHA, docosahexaenoic acid, 22:6 n-3. Although we have the enzymes that can make these long chain fatty acids from the mother of all omega 3 fatty acid, ALA, alphalinolenic acid, 18:3 n-3. It is vital to know that these polyunsaturated fatty acids as well as the omega 6 counter parts must be protected from lipid peroxidation. The very oxygen that we breath can attack the double bonds in the fatty acids and produce toxic peroxides. These peroxides are unstable and quickly decompose, breaking the chain to form toxic aldehydes. Vitamin E is the antioxidant protector of PUFA's. So, you need to take a 400 IU supplement of vitamin E with the omega 3 fatty acids. We typically get a disproportionate amount of omega 6 fatty acids in our diet, but not enough omega 3.

What do these omega 3 fatty acid supplements do for us? A supplement of 4000 mg of omega 3 fatty acids can lower triglycerides, reduces oxidized LDL's, reduces inflammation, reduces the risk of high blood pressure and irregular heartbeats. They also decrease the risk of Metabolic Syndrome and Diabetes. (Knowlton, SR. "Maximizing Omega-3 Health Benefits." Life Extension. 20:62-71. June 2014.)

The fifth recommended **supplement is Curcumin**. Curcumin is a component of the spice, turmeric. Curcumin is polyphenol that is a powerful antioxidant and anti-inflammatory supplement. Over 9,500 scientific papers are currently in the medical literature. A review of over 100 of these studies was published in 2014 with the following findings. (Aggarwal, BB. "Curcumin. A component of the Golden Spice: From Bedside to Bench and Back." Biotechnology Advances. 2014.) Curcumin blocks tumor formation by activating the P-53 and the P-21 tumor suppressor genes. It also blocks tumor growth and metastasis (spreading of the tumor). Curcumin reduces arterial inflammation preventing the oxidation of LDL's and platelet aggregation (clot formation). It protects nerve axons from

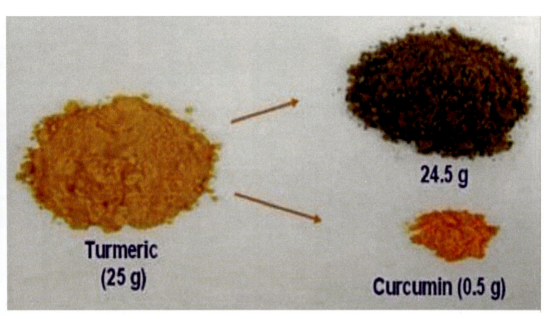

oxidative attack in M.S., multiple sclerosis), a degenerative autoimmune disease of the nervous system. It has a powerful antistress effect, stimulate the formation of new brain cells and it lowers cortisol production. (Johnston, A. "Curcumin Reverses the cellular Damage of Chronic Stress." Life Extension. 22:65-70. December 2016.)

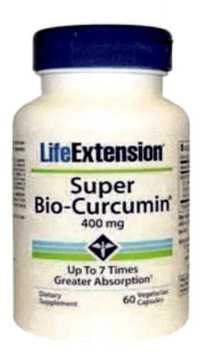

Life Extension has produced a curcumin supplement called Biocurcumin that is absorbed seven times greater than pure curcumin extract. (Iver, VS. et al. "A pilot Cross-over Study to Evaluate Human Oral Bioavailability of BCM-95CG (Biocurcumax), A Novel Bioenhanced Preparation of Curcumin." Indian Journal of Pharmacological Science. 70:445-9. 2008.)

One in four Americans will die of cancer. Cancer is a disease that turns off the Apoptotic (Death) program in cells. The resulting cells become immortal. Curcumin reverses this, turning on the death program causing sick cells to kill themselves. Curcumin modulates cell signaling mechanisms that initiate a cancer and inhibits growth factors that stimulate cancer growth. (Chen, V. "How Curcumin Targets Cancer." Life Extension. 22:44-51. September 2016.)

Curcumin increases the formation of new neurons. It helps prevent neurodegenerative diseases. It exhibits antiaging properties and acts as a powerful free radical scavenger, thus protecting DNA from mutational damage. Curcumin protects and supports the integrity of mitochondria. It turns off oncogenes (cancer causing genes) and inhibits blood flow to existing cancers. (Stevens, J. "Aging Brains and Cancer." Life Extension. 22:38-46.
March 2016.)

It has been established for over 12 years that the combination of **Acetylcarnitine and Alpha Lipoic Acid** protect mitochondria from oxidative damage. Being inside of a mitochondrion is like being in a fire in an asbestos suit or being in a room with five shooters outside peppering the room with bullets. Mitochondria need all the help they can get to protect themselves. (Ames, BN. "Delaying the mitochondrial decay of aging." Annals of the New York Academy of Science. 1019:406-11. June 2004.)

The sixth recommended **supplement is Coenzyme Q_{10}.** Coenzyme Q_{10} (CoQ) or Ubiquinone is a component of the Electron Transport System in the mitochondria of cells. This is the cellular system that produces ATP (the high-energy molecule of life). When this author was a chemistry graduate student in 1964 at Indiana University, he worked in a research laboratory with a post-doctoral student named, Charley Sharp. He was trying to discover the role that CoQ plays in the electron transport system. Fifty-two years later, we know that a decrease in CoQ causes a decrease in energy production. As energy production wanes, the cells do not have enough energy to produce the required molecules of life. This results in energy deprivation in the heart and the brain, the two most energy demanding organs in the body. This creates an energy crisis in all the cells of the body.

Research has shown that rats supplemented with CoQ had a longevity increase of 11.7%. Extrapolating to humans, having an average life span of 78.8 years, would mean that our life expectancy would increase 9 years. This is because CoQ is a powerful antioxidant, helping to squelch the massive number of free radicals produced by normal mitochondrial activity. This can result in decreasing the incidence of degenerative deceases. (Stoddard, J. "Shilajit Boosts CoQ10 Efficiency." Life E. February 2016.)

Combining supplements of 200 mg of CoQ with 200 ug of selen Extension two-a-day multi-vitamin/mineral supplement) can decrease death by 53%. A ten-year Swedish study showed that participants tha selenium/CoQ supplements displayed 49% fewer incidence of stroke, h ..tack and congestive heart failure. Studies also show that selenium improves the efficacy of CoQ supplementation. (Rogers, J. "Combining CoQ10 and Selenium Reduces Cardiovascular Mortality." Life Extension. 22:22-27. October 2016.)

Resveratrol is the seventh supplement that we are recommending. Resveratrol is a polyphenol with potent antioxidant properties. It is found in red wine, but as discussed in the former article in this book, you cannot drink enough wine to be as efficacious as one dose of supplement of 200 mg. Resveratrol promotes youthful gene expression, thus offers protection against aging. It also helps protect mitochondria from oxidative damage. It promotes a healthy insulin sensitivity which guards against diabetes. It also promotes healthy cardiovascular function, protecting arteries from atherosclerosis (the disease of the arterial surfaces leading to heart attack).

The eighth **supplement that we are recommending is PQQ, PyrroloQuinoline Quinone.** PQQ is not produced in the bodies of mammals. It is naturally produced in a variety of plants, the richest sources being parsley, green tea, kiwi, papaya, tofu (soy) and spinach. The recommended dosage is 20 mg per day. There are currently over 800 scientific papers published in the medical literature on PQQ.

Recent studies have shown PQQ to be particularly influential in mitochondria. PQQ promotes previously immortal cancer cells to self-destruct (Apoptosis) by suppressing cancer growth factors and activating mitochondrial genes that promote Apoptosis. (Cheng, Y. "PQQ Induces Cancer Cell Apoptosis via the Mitochondrial Dependent Pathway and Down Regulating Cellular Bcl-2 Protein Expression." Journal of Cancer. 5:609-624. 2014.)

PQQ has been shown to be neuroprotective and can help protect memory and cognition in the elderly. PQQ stimulates the growth of new nerve cell by activating nerve growth factors. This can stimulate the growth of new brain cells. Glutamate (an amino acid that concentrates in the brain) excess in the brain causes **excitotoxicity** which promotes brain inflammation and increased apoptosis in healthy brain cells. PQQ reverses and stops this

PQQ inhibits the formation of **beta amyloid** proteins in the brain that lead to Alzheimer's and Parkinson's Diseases. (Hopkins, C. "How PQQ Protects the Brain." <u>Life Extension.</u> 22:25-31. April 2016).

In a recent review article, PQQ was reported to have growth promoting activity, antidiabetic, antioxidant and neuroprotective effects. (Akagawa, M. "Recent progress in studies on the health benefits of pyrroloquinoline quinone." <u>Bioscience, Biotechnology, Biochemistry.</u> 80:13-22. July 13, 2015).

There are hundreds of supplements on the market, many of which have grandiose claims that are not confirmed by scientific research. Many products have not been researched at all. We have chosen to highlight the few that we actually take as part of our nutritional regimen. These supplements have been extensively researched and deemed effective. Have a Healthy Life.

CHAPTER 11 - BOGUS NUTRITION: A DISCUSSION OF CONTROVERSES

There are many bogus claims about various aspects of nutrition. We are going to explore and expose a few of these. One of the spurious claims in nutrition is the phenomenon of **FAT BURNERS**. This author wrote the following article published on EZINE.

CONTROVERSY ONE

LET'S TALK ABOUT FAT BURNERS
By Professor Jack Bateman

There are many products on the market today that offer ingredients that are advertised to "Burn Fat." Let's examine the cold, hard facts. This is going to get very technical, but it is the only way I know to expose the truth about fat burning.

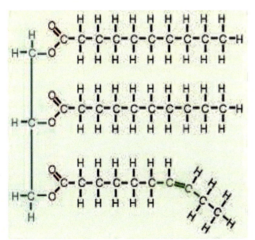

A fat molecule is called a triglyceride. It is composed of a glycerol backbone and three fatty acids, symbolized by a zigzag line. The bond that connects the glycerol to the fatty acids is called an ester bond. Enzymes call LIPASES break the ester bond during the digestion process.

3 Fatty Acids + Glycerol

LIPASE ATTACKS HERE

Your cells are composed of cell parts (organelles) that are encased in cell membrane material. Cell membranes are composed of fatty molecules called phospholipids. A phospholipid is composed of a glycerol backbone capable of bonding to three different molecules via ester bonds. Two of those bonding sites are bonded to fatty acids, which can be saturated or unsaturated. The third bonding site is a hydrophilic (water loving) phosphate that has three other bonding sites of its own. One of those bonding sites is attached to an amino alcohol called choline (typically).

A phospholipid is symbolized by an egg-shaped oval (the water-soluble choline and phosphate) with two tail like projections (the water hating fatty acids) protruding from it. Cell membranes are composed of a phospholipid bilayer with the fatty acid molecules in the middle and the phosphate groups on the inner and outer surfaces of the membranes.

The cartoon below depicts a cell membrane showing protein molecules that traverse the bilipid layer and a protein on the inner surface of the membrane. Cholesterol molecules in animal cells help stabilize the bilipid layer (plants do not make cholesterol). Carbohydrate chains on the outer surface of the membrane act like traffic cops. They attract and guide molecules to the outer surface of the membrane.

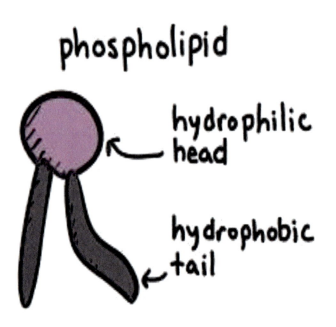

So, a cell is encased in such a membrane, as well as the organelles, like the nucleus and mitochondria.

The mitochondria have an outer membrane and an inner membrane, typical of bacteria. These membranes hold proteins that act like gates to screen what molecules get in or out of the structure, like the bean shaped cartoon below

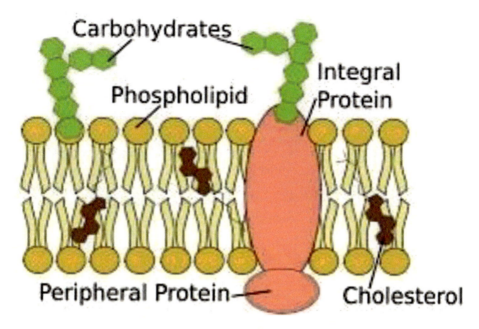

MITOCHONDRION

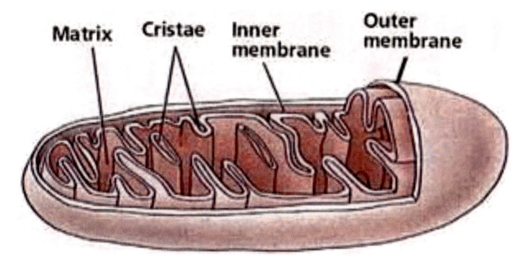

All fat is burned inside the matrix (inner membrane) of the mitochondrion. Fat or triglycerides are broken down into free fatty acids (FFA) and glycerol in the cell. Outside the mitochondrial membrane, the free fatty acids are attached to an energetic molecule called, **Coenzyme A**, which contains the B vitamin, **Pantothenic Acid** or B 5. This Co A-fatty acid complex passes through the outer membrane of the mitochondrion.

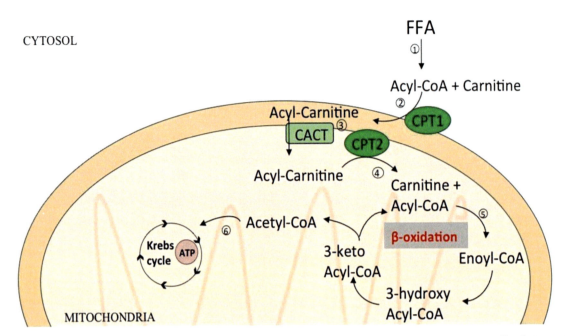

On the inner membrane of the mitochondrion it encounters an enzyme called **CARNITINE ACYLTRANSFERASE II** that exchanges the Co A for an amino acid called **CARNITINE**. The carnitine-fatty acid complex passes through the inner membrane of the mitochondrion. Once inside the matrix of the mitochondrion the fatty acid is reattached to Co Enzyme A, after which it can enter the **FATTY ACID CYCLE**. The fatty acid cycle is only found in mitochondria. The output molecules from the fatty acid cycle can be burned for energy. Remember that fat contains 2.5 times the energy of a carbohydrate.

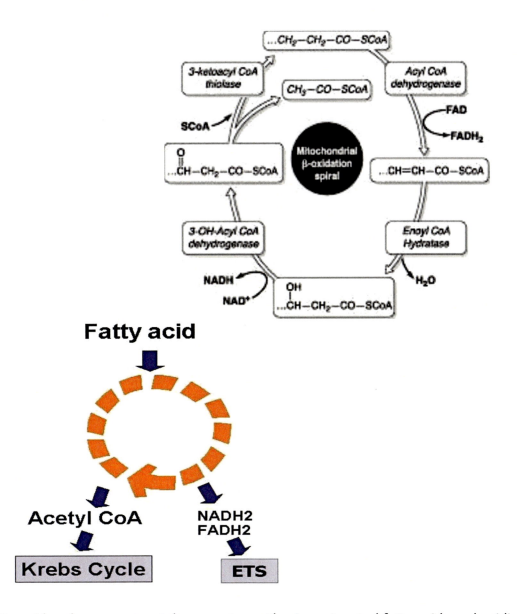

The fatty acid cycle can use acetyl groups to synthesize saturated fatty acids and oxidize saturated fatty acids breaking them down into acetyl groups. Acetyl groups are transported by Coenzyme A (CoA). Since acetyl groups contain two carbon atoms, fatty acids are broken down two carbon atoms at a time. They are also synthesized two carbon atoms at a time. Therefore, fatty acids have even numbers of carbon atoms.

What is a "FAT BURNER"? In the popular literature and advertising of either weight loss or body building genre, fat burners are substances that either increase your heart rate, mobilize fat stores, or stimulate hormone release. Many of them have side effects.

Substances like caffeine, synephrine, and yohimbine stimulate the adrenal glands to release epinephrine and nor epinephrine. These hormones act on almost every tissue in the body increasing your need for energy, so you burn more calories. Initially you burn carbohydrate followed in 15 – 30 minutes by fat mobilization and increased fat burn. So, is there a limit to the amount of fat that can be burned through chemical stimulation? The answer is yes. It depends on the concentration of mitochondria in the cells of your body, especially muscle cells. The number of mitochondria in cells is a function of aerobic exercise. One of the benefits of aerobic exercise is the stimulation of mitochondria production.

Mitochondria have their own DNA, thus can control their own rate of division and proliferation. Research has proven that aerobic exercise increases the number of mitochondria in muscle cells. **Where do we burn fat?** We burn fat in mitochondria of course. The more you have, the better you can burn fat. So, without aerobic exercise, there is a definite limit to your ability to burn fat.

Fat is stored in Adipose (FAT) cells. This fat can be released when the fat cells receive signals that activate lipolysis, lipo = fat, lysis = to break apart, (the breakdown of stored fat). The mobilized fat, now back in circulation, can either be redeposited or burned If you do not provide the exercise demand for more fat to be burned, then it will be redeposited, perhaps on your arteries.

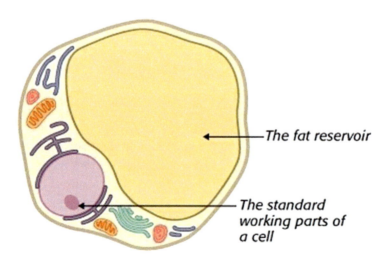

ADIPOSE CELL

Now, I ask you, does it make any sense that a supplement could magically burn fat, after seeing how complex fat burning is? Not unless it could increase the fat-carnitine transport across the mitochondrial membrane.

Fat burning DOES NOT OCCUR ANY OTHER WAY, nor in any other place in the cell.

BEWARE OF MAGICAL "FAT BURNERS". 2014.

CONTROVERSY TWO

The next questionable topic is the **GLUTEN FREE DIET.** Gluten is a protein found in many grains like wheat, rye, and barley. One percent of the population have a disease called *CELIAC DISEASE* in which gluten produces an immune response that leads to the inflammation of the digestive tract.[7] This is a serious disease that can result in severe damage to the intestinal membranes resulting in malabsorption syndrome. If your intestinal membranes are so damaged that you cannot absorb the nutrients that you eat, you develop nutritional deficiencies. The nutrients that are not absorbed pass into the colon where they feed the bacteria that reside in the colon. These colon bacteria produce waste products that irritate the colon producing an immune response that results in diarrhea. Patients that experience diarrhea day after day develop dehydration and mineral deficiencies. This condition can result in anemia, joint and bone pain abdominal bloating, skin rashes, mouth sores, anxiety, and depression. Celiac disease patients must avoid gluten completely. There are some grains that do not contain gluten, for example: Amaranth, millet, and quinoa (technically a seed).

Another group of people develop allergies to gluten. They comprise about 6 to 8% of the population. Another 10 to 20% of the population can develop a sensitivity to gluten. These conditions have led to the food manufacturers to produce a plethora of *gluten free foods*. They often label foods "Gluten Free" that could not contain gluten, just to attract buyers. These marketing practices prey on the ignorance of the general public. My hope is that this book enlightens people so that they can avoid these fool's traps. This has led to a current FAD in which many people think that they must avoid the consumption of gluten. There is a psychology behind people that gravitate to FADs. Perhaps they have a need to be included in something. There is an inherent danger in joining this FAD. By eliminating gluten from your diet, you are depriving yourself of most the available whole grains along with the fiber and micronutrients that they contain.[7] Whole grains are the principal source of insoluble fiber that promote a decrease in transit time. Decreased transit time helps prevent colon disease including colon cancer. Mitochondria are the FAT burner organelles.

[7] Koning, F. "Adverse Effects of Wheat Gluten." Annals of Nutrition & Metabolism. 67: 8-14. November 2015

CONTROVERSY THREE

The next myth to be discussed is that **brown eggs** are more nutritious than white eggs. Chemical analysis shows that there is virtually no difference in nutrient composition between the two.[8] However, if you can find eggs from range fed chickens, buy them because the egg yolks will probably be orange due to a high content of vitamin A. They will be rich in other nutrients as well. They typically contain more omega 3 fatty acids than other eggs. You can actually find omega 3 enriched eggs in the grocery. The layer chickens are fed omega 3 enriched meal and allowed to forage for wild seeds, berries and insects. This author once raised 50 chickens that were allowed to forage for food. The eggs that they laid were superior.

[8] "Are brown eggs tastier and more nutritious than white eggs?" Consumer Reports. March 2014.

CONTROVERSY FOUR

The fourth myth is the bogus claim that **eating more protein** will build muscle. Even though you need protein to build muscle, your body will not build more muscle unless you create a need. You create the need by asking muscles to do more than they have been doing in the past. It is called resistance training or weight training. The two cardinal principals are *Intensity and duration.* You should start with light weights performing 3 sets of 5-10 lifts. When the activity becomes easy, increase the weight. The more you challenge your muscles to do, the more muscle you will build and the more mitochondria you will have. Remember that there is a genetic limit to how large your muscle mass can become. Exercising your muscles to optimal strength is ideal.

CONTROVERSY FIVE

The controversy #5 is that **Organic foods** are more nutritious than non-organic foods. What does Organic food mean? The USDA (United States Department of Agriculture) sets rules and regulation for farmers wanting to do Organic Farming. They use natural fertilizers, no chemical pesticides, or fertilizers. Companion planting controls pests, meaning that there are certain plants that naturally repel a given crop pest. There are 1.7 million scientific articles currently published on this topic. The consensus is that consuming organic foods provide more nutrients and less toxins than traditionally farmed foods.³ Organic foods are usually more expensive than traditional foods, so it is a matter of choice. Can you afford the added cost to buy organically grown food? If you can, then it is wise to do so.

Pesticides and environmental toxins, like PCB's (Polychlorinated Biphenyls) are persistently in foods and the water supply, even though they have been banned for over a decade. PCB's are infinitely toxic as a mutagen (causes genetic mutations) and a carcinogen (causes cancer) as well as a neurological poison. They were banned in the U.S. in 1979 and World Wide in 2001. PCB's have a half-life of 10-15 years in the human body. The more fat you have, the more PCB's you have stored there. A half-life is the time that it takes for half of a substance to disappear. This means that you never get rid of all the substance... the whole life is infinity. Pesticides like DDT and its derivatives have half-lives of up to 37 years. They are also stored in body fat. DDT and its derivatives were banned in 1972, so it has had between two and five half-life decays. This means that we still have between 3 and 25% of it left in the environment.[4,11]

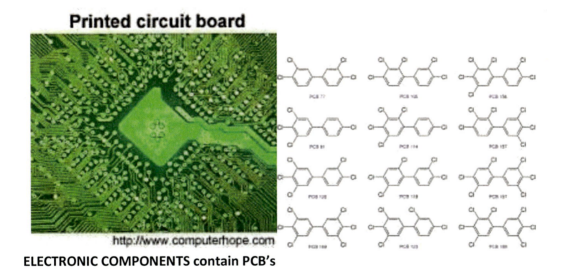

ELECTRONIC COMPONENTS contain PCB's

POLYCHLORINATED BIPHENYLS

---

[3] Crinnion, W. "Organic foods contain higher levels of certain nutrients, lower levels of pesticides, and may provide health benefits for the consumer." <u>Alternative Medicine Reviews.</u> 4:210+. October 4, 2016.

[4] Public Health Statement for DDT, DDE, and DDD. <u>Agency for Toxic Substances and Disease Registry</u>. September 2002.

The Truth About Nutrition

[11] Heinzow, B. "Elimination Half-lives of Polychlorinated Biphenyl Congeners in Children." Environmental Science and Technology. 42:6991-6996. September 15, 2008.

CONTROVERSY SIX

The 6th myth is that **saturated fat** is actually healthy for you. The truth is that you need some saturated fat to make cell membranes that are stable. The consumption of saturated fat stimulates the synthesis of cholesterol. There are 3700 medical journal articles currently published on this topic. Although there is some controversy regarding the healthy amount of saturated fat in the daily diet, there is consensus that substituting unsaturated fat for saturated fat decreases the risk of atherosclerosis and coronary artery disease, CAD.[12,13] The American Heart Association recommends that saturated fat should comprised no more that 7% of your total fat consumption per day.

As the Mediterranean pyramid shows, we need to minimize our consumption of red meats to lower our saturated fat intake. Remember that saturated fat is solid, so much so that you could literally cut the fat off a large piece of beef and use it as a weapon. When you must eat a piece of beef, try to have something with unsaturated fat with it. Instead we eat a hamburger, French fries, and a milk shake, all of which contain mostly saturated fat. We could have chosen a salad with an olive oil dressing to go with the hamburger. If you include some avocado in that salad you would have some very valuable unsaturated fat as well as a lot of micronutrients.

[12]Zock, et.al. "Progressing Insights into the Role of Dietary Fats in the Prevention of Cardiovascular Disease." Current Cardiology Reports. 111:11. November 18, 2016.

[13]Mensink, et.al. "Effects of Dietary Fatty Acids and Carbohydrates on the Ratio of Serum Lipids." American Journal of Clinical Nutrition. 77: 1146-1155. May 2003.

CONTROVERSY SEVEN

The 7th myth is that **Colon Cleansing** is necessary because "wastes, toxins and parasites" build up in our bodies leading to a range of intestinal health issues such as bloating, gas, and fatigue. Internal cleansing allows the body to rid itself of toxins and harmful wastes to promote a healthy colon and positive sense of well- being. Friends, this is a multimillion dollar industry with brick and mortar stores performing this bogus act. The truth is that your colon does not store pounds of sludge and toxic waste for long periods of time unless you are always constipated. A healthy colon gets rid of its contents in 24-48 hours. With the consumption of proper amounts of fiber, this retention time can be shortened. The use of a **probiotic supplement** can improve one's transit time. "Effective nourishment and support will optimize good colon and intestinal health, encouraging proper digestion and regular bowel movements."[14] The Mediterranean Diet provides the whole grains, vegetables and fruits necessary to consume 20-40 g of fiber per day. This will insure a healthy transit time allowing 1-2 bowel movement per day.

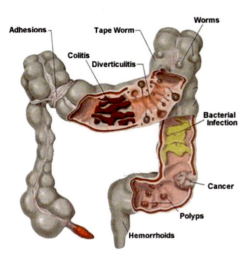

CONTROVERSY EIGHT

The 8th bogus claim is that **Canola Oil** is loaded with trans-fatty acids. A review of the medical literature found one research article that showed some trans fatty acid in canola oil. The research was done in Bogota, Columbia. There chemical analysis of various cooking oils showed that canola oil had the lowest content of trans-fatty acid at 0.4%, whereas sunflower oil had the highest content at 2.18%.[15] Not one additional research papers suggested that canola oil was contaminated with trans-fatty acid.

[14]Seow-Choen, F. "The Physiology of Colonic Hydrotherapy." Colorectal Disease. 11:686-688. September 2009.

[15]Mouynihan, M. et.al. "Trans-fatty acids in cooking oils in Bogota, Columbia: changes in the food supply from 2008-2013." Public Health Nutrition. 18: 3260-3264. December 18, 2015.

CONTROVERSY NINE

The 9th myth is that you can get all the **omega 3 fatty acids** you need by eating fish. Scientific consensus tell us that we need 2 – 3 grams of fish oil per day. Harvard's School of Public Health reports that we get the following amounts of long chain omega 3 fatty acids from the following sources:

3 oz of Anchovy	1.8 grams
6 oz of Halibut	0.79 grams
6 oz of wild Salmon	1.77 grams
6 oz of farmed Salmon	4.5 grams
6 oz of Albacore Tuna	1.46 grams

Remember that omega 3 fatty acids are used to produce omega 3 prostaglandins that counteract omega 6 prostaglandins. This is an essential balance that must occur for good health. There are only two essential fatty acids (EFA), meaning that you must have them and you cannot make them. The essential omega 3 fatty acid (EFA) is alpha linolenic acid or ALA. It can be obtained from walnuts, canola oil, some legumes, and flax seed, not from eating fish. The omega 6 EFA is linoleic Acid (LA), 18:3 Ω-6. The omega 3 fatty acids that we obtain from eating fish can be derived from ALA. They have longer chains of carbon atoms than ALA. So, the bottom line is that you need both. The chemical short hand for ALA is 18:3 Ω-3, meaning that there are 18 carbon atoms, three double bonds, the first of which is on the third carbon from the last carbon atom in the chain. From eating fish, we get 20:5 Ω-3, EPA (Eicosapentaenoic acid. Eicosa means 20 carbons, pentaen means 5 double bonds) and 22:6 Ω-3, DHA (docosahexaenoic acid, docosa means 22 carbons, hexaen means 6 double bonds). Observe that carbons are added to the fatty acid chain two at a time. This is because they come from acetyl groups that contain two carbon atoms that are the output of the fatty acid cycle.

CONTROVERSY TEN

The next controversy involves **SUGAR**. Is there evidence that sugar consumption can lead to degenerative disease? How much sugar can we safely consume? Are all sugars created equal? The consensus recommendation is that sugar should not comprise more that 10% of your daily Calorie consumption. Interestingly one 12-ounce Coca Cola contains 168 Calories of sugar. Consider a female daily Calorie intake of 1500 Calories, 10% would be 150 Calories, meaning that one 12-ounce Coke would exceed their daily maximum. One study concluded that sucrose consumption of 15% of Calories is associated with an increased risk of a cardiac event.[16] The absorption of sugar is a function of the glycemic index.[17, 18]

Glucose is the typical standard for determining the Glycemic Index (GI) of a food with a value of 100. High GI values are between 71 and 100+. High GI foods contain sugars that are rapidly absorbed, causing a large insulin response that leads to the rapid movement of glucose out of the blood stream and into the cells of the body.

[16] Barclay, A.W. "Glycemic index, glycemic load, and chronic disease risk – a meta-analysis of observational studies." American Journal of Clinical Nutrition. 87:627-37. March 2008.

[17] Diurhuus, C.B., et al. "Effects of cortisol on lipolysis and regional interstitial glycerol levels in humans." American Journal of Physiological and Endocrinological Metabolism. 283:172-7. 2001

[18] Harvard Mental Health Letter. February 2012.

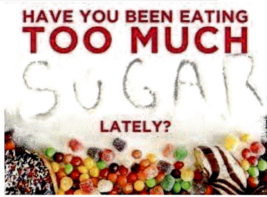
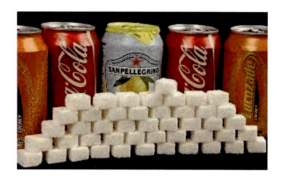

This rapid transport of glucose results in the release of **Cortisol,** a steroid hormone produced by the adrenal glands.[19] This hormone promotes the release of glucose into the blood stream that leads to a hyperglycemic event (Diabetes). Stress also causes the release of Cortisol, exacerbating the blood level which lead to immune suppression.[20] Some of the immune proteins that are inhibited are anti-tumor proteins.[21] This results in increased mutation of cancer causing genes (Oncogenes) which leads to an increase risk of cancer development.

Cortisol interferes with the activation of the GLUT 4 glucose transport mechanism in most of the cells in the body.[22] This means that glucose cannot get out of the blood stream which leads to hyperglycemia. Cortisol can influence the mobilization of fat that can lead to increased deposits on the surface of arteries causing CAD, coronary artery disease.

While performing the literature search on these topics, we discovered more than seven thousand research publication about sugar consumption and disease. There were over 173,000 publications about sugar consumption and cancer. Over 53,000 publications on heart disease and sugar appeared on PubMed. A review article concluded that the consumption of fructose, a component of sucrose (table sugar) and high fructose corn syrup presents a greater risk of coronary heart disease than does saturated fat.[23] Many other studies have proven that replacing saturated fat with unsaturated fat is very heart healthy.

After reading dozens of research reports, we must conclude that the consumption of sugar is definitely related to heart disease and cancer. We must limit of consumption to 10% of our Calorie consumption.

19. Krtolica, A. and Campisi, J. "Cancer and Aging: A model for the cancer promoting effect of the aging stroma. The International Journal of Biochemistry and Cell Biology. 34:14011414. November 2002.

20. Besedovsky, H.O. et.al. "Integration of Activated Immune Cell Products in Immune Endocrine Feedback Circuits." Progress in Leukocyte Biology. 5:200. 1986

21. Warfa, K. et.al. "Association between sucrose intake and acute coronary event risk and effect modification by lifestyle factors: Malmo Diet and Cancer Cohort Study. British Journal of Nutrition. 24: 1-10. October 2016.

22. Zazpe, I. "Association between a dietary carbohydrate index and cardiovascular disease in the SUN Project." Nutrition Metabolism and Cardiovascular Disease. 26:1048-1056. November 2016.

23. DiNicolantonio, J.J. et.al. "Evidence for Saturated Fat and Sugar Related to Coronary Heart Disease." Progress Cardiovascular Disease. 58:464-72. March-April 2016.

What can we do to minimize the risks that fat and sugar pose to our health? Clearly from the medical literature presented here, we need to minimize our consumption of sugar and saturated fat. We need to change our mindset about sweets. We do not need to have a sweet desert at every meal. Fruit is a great alternative, especially the highly-colored fruits, since they contain a wide variety of biochemicals that actually prevent cancer and other degenerative diseases. Factory foods often have an abundance of sugar added to boost sales, because the food manufacturers know that people like sweet foods. Sugary soft drinks are one of the biggest culprits. We need to minimize or eliminate our consumption of these demon drinks, even fruit juices should be minimized.

CONTROVERSY ELEVEN

The 11th controversy is **ARTIFICIAL SWEETENERS**, like **aspartame** (NutraSweet), **acesulfame K**, **sucralose** (Splenda) and **saccharin**. Aspartame is a molecule composed of two amino acids (dipeptide), aspartic acid and phenylalanine. A methyl alcohol group is attached to the acid group of aspartic acid to make an ester. When it is digested the methyl, alcohol is remove first, then the dipeptide is cleaved by the enzyme, peptidase, releasing the two amino acids. Methyl alcohol is extremely toxic. It freely crosses the blood-brain barrier where it can destroy the optic nerve.
Methyl alcohol is metabolized to formaldehyde, then on to formic acid, all of which are neurotoxic.
Aspartic acid levels elevate in the brain where it can be converted to glutamate (another amino acid) which has signaling capabilities in the brain that can cause migraine headaches.[24]

In 2014 J. Ashok reported in Redox Biology, volume 29, that aspartame caused changes in the brain chemistry that increase brain cell death (Apoptosis). In 2015 Alkafafy reported in the international Journal of Immunopathology and Pharmacology, volume 28, that their research showed that aspartame and saccharin administration in rats produced signaling changes in the liver that could produce cancer with long term exposure. The literature search produced very few research reports about saccharin. This author's advice is to use these two artificial sweeteners very sparingly.

The toxicity of the artificial sweetener, Acesulfame K, has not been researched. In the literature, several research scientists are calling for the need to research this sweetener. Grotz reported in the journal, Regulation Toxicology and Pharmacology, volume 55, October 2009, that sucralose is safe for its intended use. There were no research articles that suggested otherwise. **Neotame** is a relatively new artificial sweetener that has no reports of toxicity. It is the only artificial sweetener that is endorsed by critics. **Stevia** is another sweetener that is extracted from the Stevia leaf. It has not displayed any toxicity.

SWEETENER	SWEETENING POWER
Acesulfame K	200 X
Aspartame (NutraSweet)	200
Neotame	7,000 – 13,000 X

The Truth About Nutrition

Saccharin	300 X
Stevia (Truvia)	150 X
Sucralose (Splenda)	600 X

[24] Tandel, K.R. "Sugar substitutes: Health controversy over perceived benefits." Journal of Pharmacology and Pharmacotherapy. 2:236-43. October 2011.

There are several sugar alcohols that are used to sweeten gums and candies including Sorbitol, Xylitol, and Mannitol. They are not as sweet as sucrose, but only contribute about 2.6 Calories/g. They are generally considered safe.

CONTROVERSY TWELVE

The 12th controversy is the claim that **COCONUT OIL IS BENEFICIAL AND GOOD FOR US.** Coconut oil and Palm oil are considered Tropical oils. They are both highly saturated, coconut oil is 90% saturated and Palm oil is 50% saturated. Saturated fats have the reputation of leading to high cholesterol and fatty deposits on arteries leading to CHD, coronary heart disease. In the land of saturated fatty acids, there are distinctly three different categories. There are long chain fatty acids with 14 or more carbon atoms, medium chain fatty acids with 8 – 12 carbon atoms, and short chain fatty acids with 2 – 6 carbon atoms. The medium and short chain fatty acids can be absorbed through the intestinal membranes into the hepatic-portal blood system, whereupon they travel to the liver. Arriving in the liver as free molecules, these short and medium chain fatty acids are

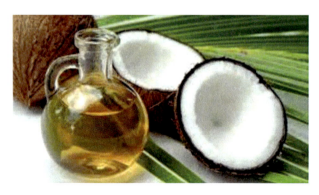

much more readily available to the fatty acid cycle than their sluggish long chain relatives.

The long chain fatty acids and monoglycerides are encumbered in large globules called chylomicrons. In the liver, chylomicrons are resynthesized into lipoprotein complexes called VLDL, Very Low Density Lipoproteins. These VLDL complexes are send into the central blood stream to be absorbed by the many cells of
the body. Even though coconut oil is 90% saturated, only 18% of the saturated fatty acids are long chain. Shorter chain and unsaturated fatty acids begin to decompose at a lower

temperature than fats that contain mostly long chain fatty acids like beef fat. Coconut oil begins to decompose at about 177°C or 350°F.

In the research review paper cited below, 8 clinical trials and 13 observational studies were reviewed. When compared to unsaturated plant oils and butter, coconut oil raised the blood level of LDL, low density lipoprotein, cholesterol more that the unsaturated plant oils, but not as much as butter. Using unsaturated oils like olive oil or canola oil lower LDL's much more and therefore, alter blood lipid profiles to reduce the risk factors for cardiovascular disease. [25]

Having reviewed the medical literature, this author would advise minimizing the use and consumption of coconut oil in favor of the unsaturated plant oils available to us. Coconut oil is consumed abundantly in the Topics, especially in less affluent countries where the availability of unsaturated plant oils is less.

[25]. Eyres, et.al. "Coconut oil consumption and cardiovascular risk factors in humans." Nutritional Reviews. 74:267-80. April 2016.

CONTROVERSY THIRTEEN

The 13th controversy is perhaps the most heated of them all. **GENETICALLY MODIFIED ORGANISMS or GMO's.** Human farmers have been preferentially selecting crop plants for over 9000 years. In 1908, George Harrison Shull described heterogenetic breeding which led to the first hybrid seed production of Maize (corn). (Wikipedia). Today almost every plant crop that is grown on a farm is a hybrid. Almost every animal that is raised on a farm or ranch is a hybrid. The hardiest specimen has been cross bred with a specimen with the most desired traits. For years, organic farmers have use companion planting and natural pesticides to increase crop productivity. One example is the use of a bacteria culture of Bacillus thuringiensis to spray on crops because when pest begin to munch on the leaves of the crop, they get sick and die. This author has used this method in his organic garden. Biotechnologists have now identified the gene that produces the protein that kills the pests. We now have the technology to transfer that gene into any crop plant rendering them resistant to some pests. The question is does that pest toxic protein have any negative effect on human that eat the crop? In most cases, WE DO NOT KNOW! Biotechnologist have identified the gene that some plants have that keep them from freezing in the winter. We can now splice that gene into the genome of cold sensitive crop plants like strawberries and oranges, which has been done. When this transgenic plant produces this antifreeze protein, does it have any effect on the human consumer? A review of the scientific literature on GMO studies finds that there is no evidence of GMO Foods harming anyone.[26,27] Several studies have been done on rats eating GMO foods compared to controls eating the same non-GMO food. Those studies have shown no ill effects from the GMO food consumption after both biochemical and anatomical analysis.[28,29]

Since the number of studies on the effects of eating GMO foods is very limited, it is clear to this author that many more studies need to be performed. It is all about time and money. While we are waiting for results from future studies, do we continue to eat GMO foods? The choice is yours.

Whereas cross breeding of farm species was performed between individuals of the same species, genetic engineering can transfer genetic information from one species to a totally different species, like the bacteria to corn.

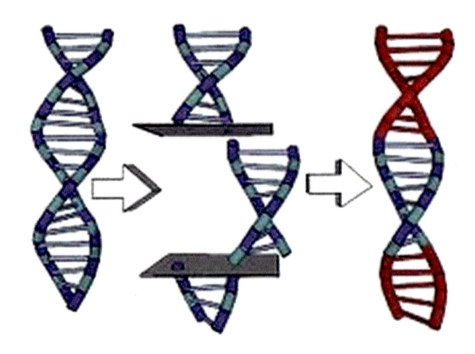

The cartoon above depicts the cutting of a double helix piece of DNA, then splicing the cut piece into a different DNA strand. With the invention of CRISPR, **C**lustered **R**egularly **I**nterspaced **S**hort **P**alindrome **R**epeats, gene alterations and transfers can occur much faster, which can lead not only to gene insertions into crops but into humans as well.[30]

References for GMO's

[26] Baklavachalam, GB, et.al. "Transgenic maize event TC1507: Global status of food, feed, and environmental safety." GM Crops and Food. 6:80-102. 2015.

[27] Guo, QY. et.al. "Effect of 90-Day Feeding of Transgenic Maize BT799 on the Reproductive System in Male Wistar Rats." International Journal of Environmental Research and Public Health. 12:15309-20. December 2, 2015.

[28] Panchin, AY. "Published GMO studies find no evidence of harm when corrected for multiple comparisons." Critical Reviews in Biotechnology. 14:1-5. January 2016.

[29] Finkelstein, PE. "Genetically Modified Foods: A Brief Overview of the Risk Assessment Process." GM Crops and Food. 18:0. February 2016 (Epub ahead of print)

[30] Maxmen, A. "Easy DNA Editing Will Remake the World." Wired. August 2015.

CONTROVERSY FOURTEEN

The 14th controversy is **IRRADIATED FOOD**, is it safe?

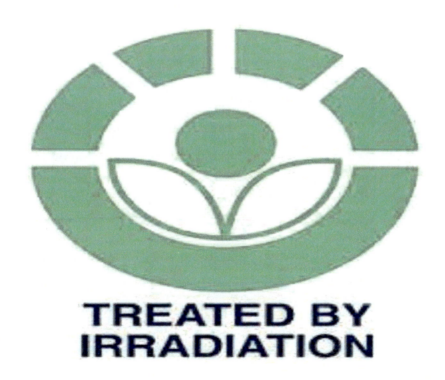

FOODS APPROVED FOR IRRADIATION IN THE USA

Approval	Food	Purpose
1963	Wheat flour	Control of mold
1964	White potatoes	Inhibit sprouting
1986	Pork	Kill Trichina parasites
1986	Fruit and vegetables	Insect control Increase shelf life
1986	Herbs and spices	Sterilization
1990 - FDA 1992 - USDA	Poultry	Bacterial pathogen reduction
1997 - FDA 1999 - USDA	Meat	Bacterial pathogen reduction

What is FOOD IRRADIATION? It is the process of exposing food to gamma rays from a radioactive source usually Cobalt – 60 or Cesium – 137. These radioactive isotopes emit high energy gamma rays that kill every living thing, including viruses, bacteria, mold, parasites, larvae, and insect eggs (almost every piece of meat you buy has fly eggs on it). The gamma rays virtually sterilize the food. Food spoils because of microorganisms attacking the food. Irradiated foods must contain the proper radiation symbol displayed on page 129.

This all sounds good until you ask what effect is the radiation having on the food itself? Gamma radiation breaks chemical bonds creating a barrage of unstable molecular fragments called **FREE RADICALS**. These molecular fragments have unpaired electrons that make them extremely reactive. They will attack every protein, fat, carbohydrate, or DNA molecule in the food. What are these newly formed chunks of biochemical molecules? There is no telling! What effects might they have on the person eating the irradiated food? We do not know in most cases; we are virtually rolling the dice. Research studies on irradiated food consumption by laboratory animals have documented some allergic effects. Chemical analysis of some foods has shown differences in the protein and carbohydrate structure after irradiation, but no adverse effects on the texture

The Truth About Nutrition

or taste of the food was noted. Research on Human consumption of gamma irradiated food is sparse at best.

Several research studies were published on irradiating bacon and the subsequent chemical analysis. When the bacon was fed to mice, no aberrant growth patterns, cancers, or other pathologies were observed. Some trace amounts of long chain hydrocarbons were observed. Roma tomatoes were irradiated with no loss of flavor or appearance. Some loss of firmness was observed.[31] The shelf life was extended for 12 days with no microbial growth.[32] In another study, Romaine lettuce was irradiated, after which no change in color, taste, or appearance when stored for 22 days. A 10% loss of firmness was observed.[33] Sesame seeds were irradiated with no effect on the quality of the lipid content. They were able to be stored for 12 months with no microbial growth. Some small changes in the protein and sugar contents were observed.[33] A final study was done on irradiating pork sausage showing that lipid oxidation was accelerated producing aldehydes, ketones, and alcohols. These products can be toxic and mutagenic leading to cancer formations.[34]

References for irradiated food.

[31] Prakash, A. et.al. "The effects of gamma irradiation on the microbiological, physical and sensory qualities of diced tomatoes." Radiation Physics and Chemistry. 63:387-390. March 2002.

[32] Prakash, A. et.al. "Effects of Low-dose Gamma Irradiation on the Shelf Life and Quality Characteristics of Cut Romaine Lettuce Packaged under Modified Atmosphere." Journal of Food Science. 65:1365. April 2000.

[33] Al-Bachir, M. "Some microbial, chemical and sensorial properties of gamma irradiated sesame (Sesamum indicum L.) seeds." Food Chemistry. 15:191-7. April 2016.

[34] Jo, C. and Ahn, DU. "Volatiles and Oxidative Changes in Irradiated Pork Sausage with Different Fatty Acid Composition and Tocopherol Content." Journal of Food Science. 1110:2621. March 2000.

MENUS - EATING BY THE MEDITERRANEAN PYRAMID

Following the Mediterranean pyramid could be a drastic change for the average American. If you want to be successful, make changes slowly. If you try to stop eating everything that you have been eating for years, your resistance to change will take over and stop you. So, drop the beef and the pork a little at a time. Cut back on your desserts a day at a time, substituting fruits and yogurt as often as possible. Give up the soft drinks a little at a time. Instead of having four a day, change to three, then two, etc. Change from white bread to whole grain bread gradually. Eventually your tastes will change so that you will prefer the new choices. Remember that you do not have to give up anything forever. When those cravings for a coke or a hamburger are overwhelming, give in and have one, just do it less frequently until it is once a month. You can help change your food choices by not buying the ones that are really bad, like soft drinks, candy, sweet rolls, donuts, sweet cereals, etc. Just do not buy them. If they are not around, you cannot eat them. It is truly a mind game.

FOOD CHOICES TO AVOID

Soft drinks, "Energy drinks"- They all contain chemicals that increase your heart rate. Not good. Whole milk – Calories in one glass = 150 with 48% of the Calories as FAT. Candy, Sweet Deserts, donuts, sweet rolls, cookies, cakes, pies, etc.

Processed meats, lunch meats, hotdogs – preserved with sodium nitrite, a carcinogen. Baloney and hotdogs are mystery meats. When I visited a meat packing factory, I was appalled to learn that the meat scraps that fell on the floor were used to make hotdogs and cheap lunch meats. Legally they are allowed to contain a limited amount of insect parts and rat feces. Let the buyer beware!

Sugary cereals – where sugar is the first or second ingredient. Refined grains foods, white bread, white pasta, white crackers, potato chips (fried) Fried foods, deep fried anything, fried chicken, fried steak, fried potatoes, etc.

FOOD CHOICES TO BE CONSUMED - Remember that variety should be optimized when making food choices. This assures that you will optimize micronutrient consumption. The following proposed menus do not specify amounts. Amounts can be chosen based on your need.

Sources of Whole grains, seeds, potatoes – 2 - 3 servings per day
Multigrain breads and pastas, Brown rice, Couscous, Quinoa, Barley, Cereals, Alfa sprouts,
Potatoes: red, Idaho baking, and white.

Sources of Fruit - 2 - 3 servings per day

Apple, Apricots, Avocado, Banana, Blue berries, Black berries, Cranberries, Dates, Raspberries, Figs, Grapefruit, Grapes, Cantaloupe, Oranges, Peach, Pear, Papaya, Pineapple, Plantains, Honeydew melon, Watermelon, Strawberries, and Tangerines.

Sources of Vegetables - 4 - 5 servings per day

Alfalfa sprouts, Amaranth leaves, Artichoke, Asparagus, Bamboo shoots, Broccoli, Brussels sprouts, Bean sprouts, Beets, Beet greens, Cabbage, Carrots, Collard greens, Green beans, Eggplant, Dark green Lettuce, various (iceberg lettuce has little nutritional value), Celery, Chickpeas, Corn, Cucumber, Hearts of Palm, Kale, Kohlrabi, Leeks, Mushrooms, Mustard greens, Potato, Olives, Onion, Peas, Snow peas, Parsley, Green pepper, Radishes, Red pepper, Yellow pepper, Hot peppers, Seaweed, Spinach, Squash (Acorn, Butternut, Spaghetti, Yellow summer, and Zucchini, Sweet Potato, Tomato, Turnips, Water chestnuts and Watercress.

Sources of Legumes and nuts - 1 – 3 servings per day

Black beans, Green beans, Kidney beans, Garbanzo beans, bean sprouts, Hummus, Black-eyed peas, Green peas, Green beans, Lima beans, Lentils, Baked beans, and Great Northern beans, Sunflower seeds, Pumpkin seeds, Sesame seeds, Almonds, Brazil nuts, Cashews, Chestnuts, Hazelnuts, Macadamia nuts, Peanuts, Peanut butter, Pecans, Pine nuts, Pistachio nuts, Walnuts, other nut butters.

Sources of Dairy - At least one serving per day. Cheese, Yogurt.

Foods to be eaten WEEKLY.

Fish and Seafood, Poultry, Eggs, Sweets.

Foods to be consumed once or twice per MONTH. Beef, Pork, Lamb, Buffalo, Venison.

The Truth About Nutrition

MENUS

awberries
anana Oatmeal
s.

Fiber-one cereal with pecans and cut peaches
Raisin bran cereal with walnuts and raspberries
Fiber-one cereal and yogurt with cashews and pear slices

Other Fruits that can be served for breakfast.

Pineapple - eat often. It contains a protein digestion enzyme called bromelain. Orange, Grapefruit, Cherries, Apples, Cantaloupe, Honeydew melon, Tangerines, and Watermelon.

Eggs – eaten once or twice a week

Eggs, poached with turkey bacon and whole grain toast
Egg omelet with cheddar cheese, mushrooms, onion, and red pepper
Egg omelet with swiss cheese, onion, avocado
Egg omelet with cut broccoli, onion, green pepper, tomato

BETWEEN MEAL SNACKS

Yogurt, nuts, raw vegetables, fruit. Raw vegetables can be cut up and stored in plastic bags or other containers for convenience. Fruits can be packaged similarly. Peanut butter on whole grain crackers.

LUNCH MENUS served with a glass of wine (Adults only)

Salad made with spinach, kale, Romaine lettuce, mushrooms, pecans, mandarin oranges, dried cranberries, and cheese chunks with a citrus dressing.

Cheddar cheese with whole grain bread covered with avocado. Blue berries, walnuts, and cut celery.

Raw, cut broccoli, kohlrabi, Portobello mushrooms, snow peas, red and yellow peppers, zucchini. Vegetable dip made with yogurt blended with either blue berries, orange, raspberries, or pineapple. Change fruits for variety. Served with whole wheat crackers and peanut butter.

Half of an avocado stuffed with a mixture of cheese chunks, garbanzo beans, grapes, and celery chunks. Served with multigrain crackers.

Brown rice with black beans season to taste. Salad with spinach, mushrooms, peas, tomato, and walnuts with a vinaigrette dressing. Cut cantaloupe with black berries.

Quinoa mixed with black beans, walnuts, onion, cut celery. Fruit salad containing apples, pears, banana, blue berries, grapes, and orange slices.

Quinoa with mushrooms, onion, baby kale, red and green peppers, garbanzo beans. Cantaloupe with grapes and macadamia nuts.

Chili with Tofu, kidney beans, black beans, onion, tomatoes, and mushrooms. Served with multigrain bread with cashew butter.

Whole wheat linguini with tomato sauce, mushrooms, and onion. Salad containing Romaine lettuce, kale, chickpeas, green pepper, cashews, and olives.

Chicken salad with onion, celery, walnuts, and mayonnaise with spinach leaves on mixed grain bread.

Avocado stuffed with Tuna salad made with onion, celery, pickle relish, mayonnaise and cut baby kale leaves. Whole grain crackers.

Raw vegetable plate containing; broccoli, cauliflower, snow peas, baby carrots, red and yellow pepper slices, cherry tomatoes, Kohlrabi strips, with hummus and multigrain crackers. Tangerines slices with yogurt.

Stir fried vegetables using a rounded skillet or wok. Start with the densest choices like broccoli, onion, 2-3 garlic cloves cauliflower, carrots, celery, sweet potato strips. All the dense vegetable should be cut into equivalent sizes. Add 1-2 oz. of olive oil to the bottom of cooking vessel. Using medium-high heat, add the dense vegetables gently moving them in and out of the intense heat using a wooden spoon. Seasonings can be added at this point. Try some "Spike" (a commercial mix of dried spices). Be creative and experimental with the addition of spices. Usually a small amount will be sufficient. Low sodium soy sauce is a nice addition. As the dense vegetables begin to soften, add a variety of the following: mushrooms, alfalfa sprouts, bean sprouts, peas, snow peas, hearts of palm, cut asparagus, parsley, watercress, bamboo shoots, water chestnuts, walnuts, almonds, and pecans. Continue to constantly move the mix in and out of the intense heat. When the color of the green vegetables reaches a maximum intensity, remove the cooking vessel from the heat. Serve over brown rice or Quinoa. This can be a dinner as well. Occasionally you can add some cooked pieces of chicken.

DINNER MENUS - Served with a glass of wine (adults only). Each menu has attempted to include a grain with either a meat or a legume for complete protein (contains all essential amino acids).

Brown rice, black beans, collard greens, beets, papaya slices, and pineapple.

Whole wheat spaghetti, ground turkey and tomato sauce with onion and red peppers. Top with parmesan cheese. Romaine lettuce salad with baby kale, tomato, yellow pepper, radishes and green onions, cantaloupe with blueberries.

Quinoa, red beans, Brussels sprouts with cheese sauce, spinach salad with mushrooms, cashews, and sunflower seeds with a citrus dressing. Sliced peaches with vanilla ice cream.

Lentils cooked with barley, onion, celery, kale, parsley, and mushrooms in chicken broth. Baked acorn squash cooked with cinnamon and brown sugar. Bananas and blackberries.

Lentils cooked with onion, celery, and kale. Stuff into a whole grain pita with spinach and cheese. Stewed apples with cinnamon.

Baked Potato stuffed with cheese, broccoli, peas, and diced onion with yogurt. Spinach salad with almonds, bean sprouts and a vinaigrette dressing. Honey dew melon stuffed with blueberries, and raspberries.

Couscous with yogurt, pine nuts, spinach, garbanzo beans, snow peas and walnuts.

Whole wheat linguini with an alfredo, clam sauce. Romaine lettuce, tomato, bean sprouts with a Caesar dressing. Strawberries and pineapple.
Chicken, broiled with sweet potato, Brussels sprouts roasted with fresh garlic and cheese sauce, apricots, and yogurt.

Salmon, broiled with lime and dill. Scalloped potatoes with cheddar cheese. Baby kale and spinach salad with a tropical dressing

Shrimp with mushrooms and snow peas on couscous. Fresh broccoli with cheese sauce. Dried cranberries, chopped walnuts and blueberries with yogurt.

INDEX

Acetylcarnitine	108
Adipose cells	27
Anabolism	60
Animal Fat Composition	87
Artificial sweeteners	124
Atherosclerosis	31, 89
ATP	12, 61
ATP CYCLE	64
Basal Metabolic Rate	66
Benefits of Aerobic Exercise	67
Best Choices for protein	39
Bile	52
Brown Eggs	118
Calcium	84, 105
Canola oil	121
Carbohydrates	12
Carnitine	114
Catabolism	61
Cell Membranes	26
Cell Structure	66
Choices of Protein	39
Cholesterol	31, 44, 53
Chromosomes	64
Coconut oil	122
Coenzyme (Q-10)	72, 93, 108
Coenzyme	60
Colon Cancer	19
Colon Cleansing	121
Colon	56
Cortisol	123
Curcumin	107

Deaminase or Transaminase	97
Diabetes	15
Dietary oils	29
Digestion	46
Digestion in the jejunum	54
Digestive processes	54
Digestive Tract	50, 52
Diverticula, Diverticulitis	57
DNA	34, 64
Duodenum	50, 52
Electron Transport	71, 93
Energy balance	69
Enzymes in Food	46
Essential Amino Acids	34, 37, 38
Essential Fatty Acids	28
Extra Virgin Olive Oil	5
Factory Foods	1
Fat Burners	111
Fat content of various foods	89
Fatty Acid Cycle	115
Fiber content of various foods	85
Fiber	19, 57
Fish	42, 43
Flaxseed	28
Food Irradiation	129
Food Labels	22
Food Pyramids	3, 4
Foods to Avoid	132
Free Radical	2, 130
Functions of Protein	36
Gastric Juice	47
Genetically modified organisms	127
GERD	49
Glucagon	14
Gluconeogenesis	22
Glucose Tolerance Test	14

Glut 4 glucose transport system	71
Gluten	44, 117
Glycemic Index	14, 17
Glycogen	12
Gout	100
Grain Comparison	76
Heart Burn	49
HDL	60
Homeostasis	14
Hyperglycemia	13
Ileum	56
Insoluble Fiber	19
Insulin	12
Irradiated Food	129
Jejunum	54
Krebs Cycle	92
LDL	90
Lipids	30
Lipids in Food Chart	30
Lipoic Acid	108
Magnesium	104
Man's Menu	9
Mediterranean Pyramid	4
Mediterranean daily menus	8, 9, 77
MENUS	132
Metabolic hormones	68
METABOLISM	59
Micronutrients Chart	73
Milk Comparisons	83
Mitochondria	92, 113
Messenger RNA	34
Niacin	62
Nitrogen balance	98
Non-essential amino acids	96
Normoglycemia	13
Nutrient Density	40

Omega 3 Fatty Acids	27
Omega 3 Supplements	122
Omega 6 Fatty Acids	27
Omega 9 Fatty Acids	27
Organic Foods	118
Pancreatic Juice	50
Peristalsis	54
Phospholipid	25
Plant Protein Sources	38
Polyphenols	5
PQQ	109
Prostaglandins	28, 30
Protein Denaturation	35
Protein Efficiency	38
Protein Nutrient Density	39
Protein	33, 118
RDAs	78
Resistance Training	67
Resveratrol	6, 109
Riboflavin	61
Saturated Fat	24, 120
Soluble Fiber	19
Sources of B-6, 9, & 12	97
Stomach	48
Structure of Proteins	35
Sugar	122
Target Heart Rate	67
Trans Fatty Acids	31
Transit Time	19, 49
Typical American Menu	10, 11
Ulcers	49
Unsaturated Fat	24
Urea	38
Villi	55
Vitamin/mineral supplements	103
VLDL	90
Whole Grain	76

Willett Food Pyramid	3
Wine	6
Woman's Menu	8

Made in the USA
Middletown, DE
16 April 2017